Herbal Medicine: Back to the Future

(Volume 6)

Infectious Diseases

Edited by

Atta-ur-Rahman ***FRS***
Honorary Life Fellow
Kings College
University of Cambridge
England
UK

&

Ka Bian
George Washington University
School of Medicine
Washington
USA

Herbal Medicine Back to the Future

(Volume 6)

Infectious Diseases

Editors: Atta-ur-Rahman, *FRS* & Ka Bian

ISSN (Online): 2542-999X

ISSN (Print): 2542-9981

ISBN (Online): 978-981-5256-32-1

ISBN (Print): 978-981-5256-33-8

ISBN (Paperback): 978-981-5256-34-5

First published in 2024.

Bentham Science Publishers Pte. Ltd.
80 Robinson Road #02-00
Singapore 068898
Singapore
Email: subscriptions@benthamscience.net

CONTENTS

PREFACE

Herbal Medicine: Back to the Future presents expert reviews on the applications of herbal medicines (including Ayurveda, Traditional Chinese Medicines, and alternative therapies) for health benefits. This series of volumes was initiated under the co- Editorship and guidance of late Prof. Ferid Murad who passed away recently. His monumental contributions to science, particularly the role of nitric oxide in health snd well being, will always be remembered. He is greatly missed.

This volume demonstrates the use of sophisticated methods to explore traditional medicine while providing readers with a glimpse into the future of herbal medicine. The book should prove to be a valuable resource for pharmaceutical scientists and postgraduate students seeking updated and critically important information regarding natural product chemistry and the pharmacology of natural materials in the treatment of infectious diseases. The chapters are written by eminent experts in the field.

Leitão *et al.*, in Chapter 1, highlights the possible application of compounds isolated from Siparuna species as antiviral agents. In Chapter 2, Vadia *et al.*, emphasise the use of Indian spices and explore their key antimicrobial components for their antibacterial activity and modes of action. Chaughule and Barve in the next chapter discuss the role of herbal medicines in the treatment of infectious diseases. Singh *et al.*, in Chapter 4, focus on the traditional approach to treating infections. In the last chapter of the book, Nawaz *et al.* explore the therapeutic potential of medicinal plants for rheumatoid arthritis. Some important plants that show antioxidant and anti-inflammatory properties against rheumatoid arthritis are discussed in this chapter.

We hope that the readers involved in the study of infectious diseases will again find these reviews valuable and thought-provoking so that they may promote further research on herbal medicines and alternative therapies.

We are grateful for the timely efforts made by the editorial personnel, especially Mr. Mahmood Alam (Editorial Director), and Ms. Asma Ahmed (Senior Manager Publications), at Bentham Science Publishers for the publication of this book.

Atta-ur-Rahman, *FRS*
Kings College
University of Cambridge
Cambridge
UK

&

Ka Bian
George Washington University
School of Medicine
Washington
USA

List of Contributors

Attya Bhatti	Department of Healthcare Biotechnology, Atta-ur-Rahman School of Applied Biosciences, National University of Sciences and Technology, Islamabad, Pakistan
Ammara Arif	Department Of Healthcare Biotechnology, Atta-ur-Rahman School of Applied Biosciences, National University of Sciences and Technology, Islamabad, Pakistan
Bhanu Pratap Singh	Department of Pharmacy, University of Kota, Kota-324005, Rajasthan, India
Carla M. Leal	Programa de Pós-graduação em Biotecnologia Vegetal e Bioprocessos (PBV), Universidade Federal do Rio de Janeiro, RJ, Brazil
Deeksha Singh	E. S. I. Hospital, Kota-324005, Rajasthan, India
Diégina A. Fernandes	Instituto de Pesquisas de Produtos Naturais (IPPN), Universidade Federal do Rio de Janeiro, RJ, Brazil
Gilda G. Leitão	Instituto de Pesquisas de Produtos Naturais (IPPN), Universidade Federal do Rio de Janeiro, RJ, Brazil
Hafiza Ayesha Nawaz	Department Of Healthcare Biotechnology, Atta-ur-Rahman School of Applied Biosciences, National University of Sciences and Technology, Islamabad, Pakistan
Jalpa Sanandia	Department of Pharmaceutical Sciences, Saurashtra University, Rajkot, Gujarat, India
Mousmi Patel	Department of Pharmaceutical Sciences, Saurashtra University, Rajkot, Gujarat, India
Nasir Vadia	Department of Pharmaceutical Sciences, Faculty of Health Sciences, Marwadi University, Rajkot, Gujarat, India
Nidhi	Department of Pharmacy, University of Kota, Kota-324005, Rajasthan, India
Rajesh S. Barve	Department of Repertory, Virar Homeopathic Medical College, Virar East, Maharashtra, 401303, India
Ramesh S. Chaughule	Department of Chemistry, Ramnarain Ruia Autonomous College, Matunga, Mumbai 400019, India
Rosineide Costa Simas	Escola de Engenharia, Universidade Presbiteriana Mackenzie, SP, Brazil
Suzana G. Leitão	Faculdade de Farmácia, Universidade Federal do Rio de Janeiro, RJ, Brazil
Uttam Singh Baghel	Gurukul Pharmacy College, Ranpur, Kota – 325003, Rajasthan, India Department of Pharmacy, University of Kota, Kota-324005, Rajasthan, India

CHAPTER 1

Brazilian *Siparuna* Species as a Source of Antiviral Agents

Carla M. Leal[1], Diégina A. Fernandes[2], Rosineide Costa Simas[3], Suzana G. Leitão[4] and **Gilda G. Leitão[2,*]**

[1] *Programa de Pós-graduação em Biotecnologia Vegetal e Bioprocessos (PBV), Universidade Federal do Rio de Janeiro, RJ, Brazil*

[2] *Instituto de Pesquisas de Produtos Naturais (IPPN), Universidade Federal do Rio de Janeiro, RJ, Brazil*

[3] *Escola de Engenharia, Universidade Presbiteriana Mackenzie, SP, Brazil*

[4] *Faculdade de Farmácia, Universidade Federal do Rio de Janeiro, RJ, Brazil*

Abstract: Influenza is an acute viral infection of the respiratory tract caused by the *Alphainfluenzavirus* whose subtypes were responsible for historical pandemics. Recently, the coronavirus SARS-CoV-2 has also affected the world, causing acute respiratory syndrome, thus rendering the search for anti-influenza and anti-SARS-CoV-2 compounds an urgent task. Plants of the genus *Siparuna* are used in Brazilian folk medicine for treating colds, fever, headaches, and rheumatic pain as well as gastrointestinal disorders. *S. apiosyce* ("Limão Bravo") is mentioned in the first Brazilian Pharmacopeia due to its importance as an ingredient in syrup and cough drops. Alkaloids, methylated and glycosylated flavonoids stand out as secondary metabolites described for these species, being also well described in the literature for their antiviral activity. During our investigation of Brazilian plants active against viral infections, the anti-influenza activity of five Amazonian *Siparuna* (*S. cristata*, *S. decipiens*, *S. glycycarpa*, *S. reginae* and *S. sarmentosa*) were investigated, showing the *n*-butanol extracts of *S. glycycarpa* and *S. sarmentosa* as the most active. Dereplication of these extracts pointed alkaloids, *O*- and *C*-glycosylated flavonoids as well as dihydrochalcones and a procyanidin dimer as potential active metabolites. On the other hand, the dichloromethane extract from *S. cristata* containing methylated flavonoids was able to inhibit the *in vitro* replication of SARS-CoV-2, where it was shown that retusin and kumatakenin presented a higher selectivity index than lopinavir/ritonavir and chloroquine controls. Further *in-silico* studies showed the potential interaction between these flavonoids and the virus proteases 3CLpro and PLpro. Here we highlight the possible application of compounds isolated from *Siparuna* species as antiviral agents.

* **Corresponding author Gilda G. Leitão:** Instituto de Pesquisas de Produtos Naturais (IPPN), Universidade Federal do Rio de Janeiro, RJ, Brazil; E-mail: ggleitao@ippn.ufrj.br

Atta-ur-Rahman & Ka Bian (Eds.)

Keywords: Alkaloids, Flavonoids, Influenza A(H1N1), Kumatakenin, Retusin, SARS-CoV-2, Siparunaceae.

1. INTRODUCTION

Several chronic and acute diseases in both humans and animals may be caused by viral infections such as dengue, influenza, measles, severe acute respiratory syndrome (SARS), and West Nile virus outbreaks [1]. Several viral diseases *e.g.* acquired immunodeficiency and respiratory syndromes, as well as hepatitis are still associated with high morbidity and mortality rates in humans around the world, despite all the progress made by Medicine in the last years [2]. The lack of effective therapies and/or vaccines for several viral infections, allied to the fast emergence of new drug-resistant viruses has made the need for new and effective chemotherapeutic agents an urgent one to treat viral diseases [3].

Natural products from plants or other organisms offer a large array of structurally diverse chemical compounds that could serve as antivirals, some of which have been shown to have great potential as drug candidates in preclinical and clinical trials. Many potentially useful medicinal plants and herbs are yet to be evaluated for further applications as therapeutic agents against diverse virus families [3 - 5].

In this context, we can highlight the Siparunaceae family, represented by two genera: *Glossocalyx* Benth and *Siparuna* Aublet. *Glossocalyx,* with 70 species is native to West Africa and occurs in shady primary forests and along roadsides. *Siparuna* is composed of 72 species occurring from Mexico to the north of South America, Bolivia, and Paraguay and is recognized in the field by its citrus smell. In general, shrubs are dioecious plants that occur in Central America and the Andes, while monoecious plants are large trees (about 15 species) that occur in the Amazon basin [6, 7]. So far, *Siparuna* is the genus with the largest number of reported studies, and a comprehensive review of its chemistry and biological activities was recently published [8].

Species of *Siparuna* occur in tropical and subtropical regions of the Southern hemisphere, with Brazil being considered a center of diversity for harboring these species in all its biomes. Plants of this genus are used in folk and traditional indigenous medicines in both South and Central America for treating colds, fever, headache, and rheumatic pain as well as gastrointestinal disorders [7, 9, 10]. The heated bark of *S. sessiliflora* and *S. thecaphora* is used to accelerate the healing of herpes sores, while the leaves of *S. guajalitensis* and *S. schimpffii* are used in tea preparation to help with fatigue [7].

Siparuna brasiliensis (synonymy: *S. apiosyce*) is a popular medicine in Brazil where it is usually called "limão bravo" and "negramina". A monograph on this plant species was included in the first Brazilian Pharmacopoeia (1926), due to its importance as an ingredient in syrup and cough drops sold by pharmaceutical companies in the past [10]. Given these facts, *Siparuna* species may be a potential source of antiviral compounds [8, 11, 12].

2. BRAZILIAN *SIPARUNA* SPECIES

2.1. Occurrence

Approximately 47 species of the genus *Siparuna* occur in the Brazilian territory, distributed in five different biomes: the Amazon, Caatinga, Pantanal, the Atlantic Forest and Cerrado. The epicenter of occurrence is in the Amazon region, where the genus comprises the great majority of species as shrubs and small trees (Fig. **1**) [7, 13].

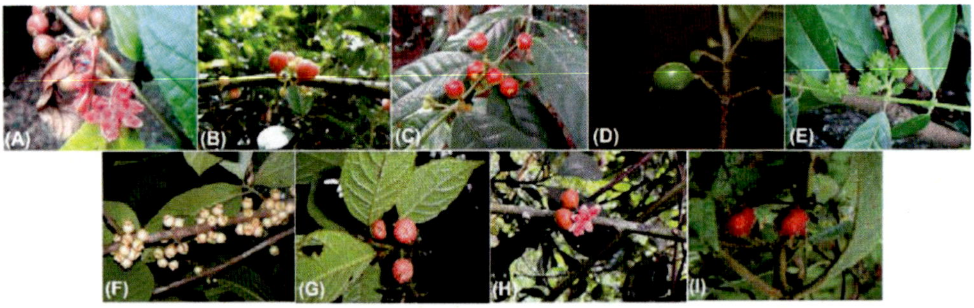

Fig. (1). *Siparuna* plants: **(A)** *S. brasiliensis*, **(B)** *S. thecaphora*, **(C)** *S. guianensis*, **(D)** *S. decipiens*, **(E)** *S. reginae*, **(F)** *S. pauciflora*, **(G)** *S. grandiflora*, **(H)** *S. lepidota* and **(I)** *S. echinata*. Source: https://www.gbif.org/species/4893899

2.2. An Overview on the Chemistry of *Siparuna*

Among the classes of secondary metabolites present in nature, free and glycosylated flavonoids with kaempferol and quercetin aglycones, aporphine and benzylisoquinoline alkaloids, and terpenoids have been previously reported in the genus *Siparuna* (Table **1,** Fig. **2**) [7 - 10]. The composition of the essential oils of many *Siparuna* species has been the aim of several studies reported in the literature as can be seen in Table **2**, showing that mono and sesquiterpenes are the major identified compounds, occurring either as hydrocarbons of common structural types (*e.g.* elemene, caryophyllene, cubebene, copaene, germacrene *etc* series) or as alcohol derivatives of these skeletal types. The flavonoid 3,7,4'-tri-*O*-methyl-kaempferol (Fig. **2**) from leaves and bark of *S. apiosyce* (*S. brasiliensis*), was the first report of an *O*-methyl flavonoid aglycone in the genus *Siparuna* [9], followed by the report of the same compound in *S. gigantotepala* [14] and *S. guianensis* [15], as well as other *O*-methylated aglycones in *S. cristata*

(3,3',4'-tri-*O*-methyl quercetin, retusin and kumatakenin, this latter being also reported for *S. gigantotepala*) [11]. Two chalcone derivatives (2',6'-dihydroxy-4,4'-di-*O*-methyl-dihydrochalcone and 2',6'-dihydroxy-4'-*O*-methyl-dihydro-chalcone) have been described until now only in the leaves of *S. glycycarpa* [12, 16, 17]. Liriodenine, an oxoaporphyne alkaloid (Fig. **2**), has been found in different species of *Siparuna*, and its presence in the leaves of *S. brasiliensis* may be responsible for its use as an antitussive medicine [7].

2.3. An Overview of Biological Activities Described for *Siparuna*

Some biological activities have been described for extracts of different polarities of several *Siparuna* species, focusing on *in vivo* and *in vitro* antimicrobial (including antifungal) and antiparasitic (antimalarial, antiplasmodial, leishmanicidal and tripanocidal) assays. Larvicidal activities, as well as anthelmintic, antioxidant, anticholinesterase and cytotoxicity against cancer cells, are also reported. Furthermore, anti-inflammatory and antiviral activities are reported for extracts from plants of this genus [8, 11, 12, 40].

Table 1. Alkaloids, flavonoids and other chemical compounds reported in the genus *Siparuna*.

Compounds	*Siparuna* Species	Plant Part	Refs.
	Alkaloids		
(+)-11-methoxy-Nomeolistine	*S. guianensis*	Leaves	[18]
Actinodaphnine	*S. decipiens*, *S. guianensis*	Leaves	[12, 18]
Ajmaline	*S. sessiliflora*	Leaves	[19]
Apoglaziovine	*S. glycycarpa*	Leaves	[12]
Annonaine	*S. glycycarpa*, *S. grandiflora*, *S. guianensis*	Leaves, stem bark, roots, stem wood, fruit	[9, 12, 20, 21]
Asimilobine	*S. brasiliensis**, *S. gesnerioides*, *S. grandiflora*, *S. guianensis*, *S. sessiliflora*	Aerial parts, stem bark, roots, fruit	[9, 10, 19, 21, 22]
Boldine	*S. cristata*, *S. decipiens*, *S. pauciflora*, *S. sarmentosa*	Leaves	[12, 18, 23]
Bulbocapnine	*S. guianensis*, *S. sarmentosa*	Leaves	[12]
Caaverine	*S. sarmentosa*	Leaves	[12, 18]

(Table 1) cont.....

Compounds	*Siparuna* Species	Plant Part	Refs.
Cassamedine	*S. guianensis*	Stem wood	[9, 20]
Cassythine	*S. sarmentosa*	Leaves	[12]
Coclaurine	*S. decipiens, S. glycycarpa, S. reginae, S. sarmentosa*	Leaves	[12, 17]
Coridine	*S. pachyantha*	Leaves	[18]
Corlumine	*S. sessiliflora*	Leaves	[19]
Dicentrine	*S. cristata*	Leaves	[12]
Demethylcoclaurine	*S. glycycarpa*	Leaves	[17]
Flavinantine	*S. dresslerana*	Leaves	[9, 24]
Fuseine	*S. guianensis*	Stem wood	[20]
Isocorydine	*S. gesnerioides, S. grandiflora*	Stem bark, roots	[9]
Isopiline	*S. glycycarpa*	Leaves	[17]
Isocorypalmine	*S. glycycarpa*	Leaves	[17]
Laurolitsine	*S. reginae, S. sarmentosa*	Leaves	[12]
Laurotetanine	*S. brasiliensis, S. grandiflora, S. pauciflora*	Stem bark, roots, leaves	[9, 10, 23]
Liriodenine	*S. brasiliensis, S. grandiflora, S. guianensis, S. pachyantha, S. poeppigii, S. thecaphora*	Leaves, stem bark, roots, stem wood, fruit, branch	[9, 10, 18, 20, 21, 24, 25]
Lysicamine	*S. poeppigii*	Leaves	[18]
Magnocurarine	*S. glycycarpa*	Leaves	[17]
N-Methyl-coclaurine	*S. glycycarpa*	Leaves	[12, 17]
N-Methyl-laurotetanine	*S. brasiliensis, S. cristata, S. gesnerioides, S. grandiflora, S. guianensis, S. pauciflora*	Stem bark, roots, fruit	[9, 10, 12, 21, 23]
N-Methyl-lindcarpine	*S. guianensis*	Leaves	[18]
N-Nornuciferine	*S. decipiens, S. glycycarpa, S. poeppigii*	Leaves	[17, 18]

(Table 1) cont.....

Compounds	*Siparuna* Species	Plant Part	Refs.
Nantenine	*S. cristata, S. gesnerioides, S. grandiflora, S. guianensis, S. pauciflora*	Leaves, stem bark, roots, fruit	[9, 12, 21]
Norboldine	*S. pauciflora*	Leaves	[23]
Norcoclaurine	*S. glycycarpa, S. sarmentosa*	Leaves	[12]
Norglaucine	*S. guianensis*	Fruit	[21]
Nornantenine	*S. grandiflora, S. guianensis*	Stem bark, roots,	[9, 21]
Norneolitsine	*S. reginae*	Leaves	[12]
Noroliveroline	*S. pauciflora*	Stem	[9]
O-Methyl-flavinanthine	*S. dresslerana*	Leaves	[9, 24]
O-Methyl-isopiline	*S. glycycarpa, S. poeppigii*	Leaves	[17, 18]
Oxonantenine	*S. grandiflora, S. thecaphora*	Stem bark, roots	[9, 24, 25]
Reticuline	*S. brasiliensis, S. cristata, S. decipiens, S. glycycarpa, S. grandiflora, S. reginae*	Leaves, stem bark, roots	[9, 10, 12, 17]
Reticuline *N*-oxide	*S. glycycarpa*	Leaves	[17]
Roemerine	*S. pachyantha*	Leaves	[18]
Stepholidine	*S. glycycarpa*	Leaves	[17]
Talicarpine	*S. sessiliflora*	Leaves	[19]
Xylopine	*S. sarmentosa*	Leaves	[12]
Amides			
cis-N-feruloyltyramine	*S. brasiliensis*	Stem bark	[10]
trans-N-feruloyltyramine	*S. brasiliensis*	Stem bark	[10]
Dihydrochalcones			
2',6'-Dihydroxy-4,4'-di-*O*-methyl-dihydrochalcone	*S. glycycarpa*	Leaves	[12, 16, 17]
2',6'-Dihydroxy-4'-*O*-methyl-dihydrochalcone	*S. glycycarpa*	Leaves	[12, 17]

(Table 1) cont.....

Flavonoids aglycones			
Retusin	*S. cristata*	Leaves	[11]
3,3',4'-tri-*O*-methyl-quercetin	*S. cristata*	Leaves	[11]
3,7,4'-tri-*O*-methyl-kaempferol	*S. brasiliensis, S. gigantotepala S. guianensis*	Leaves, stem bark	[9, 10, 14, 15]
Kumatakenin	*S. cristata, S. gigantotepala, S. guianensis*	Leaves	[11, 12, 14, 15]
Kaempferol	*S. guianensis*	Leaves	[26]
Quercetin	*S. gigantotepala, S. guianensis*	Leaves	[14, 26]
B-type procyanidin dimer	*S. guianensis, S. sarmentosa*	Leaves	[12, 27]
***O*-Glycosylated flavonoids**			
Kaempferol 3-*O*-β-glucopyranoside	*S. glycycarpa*	Leaves	[16, 17]
Kaempferol 3-*O*-β-rhamnopyranoside	*S. glycycarpa*	Leaves	[16]
Kaempferol 3-*O*-rutinoside	*S. gigantotepala, S. glycycarpa*	Leaves	[14, 17]
Kaempferol 3-*O*-glycoside-7-*O*-rhamnoside	*S. glycycarpa*	Leaves	[12, 17]
Kaempferol 3,7-di-*O*-rhamnoside	*S. guianensis*	Leaves	[27]
Kaempferol 3,7-di-*O*-methyl-4'-*O*-rutinoside	*S. gigantotepala*	Leaves	[14]
***O*-Glycosylated flavonoids**			
Kaempferol 3-*O*-hexoside-*O*-deoxyhexoside-*O*-pentoside	*S. glycycarpa*	Leaves	[17]
Kaempferol 3-*O*-pentosyl-pentoside-7-*O*- rhamnoside	*S. guianensis*	Leaves	[27]
Kaempferol 3-*O*-β-xylopyranosyl-(1→-)-α-arabinofuranoside	*S. gigantotepala*	Leaves	[14]
Kaempferol 3,7-di-*O*-methyl-4'-*O*-α-rhamnopyranos-l-(1→2)-β-gluco pyranoside	*S. gigantotepala*	Leaves	[14]
Quercetin 7-*O*-rutinoside	*S. glycycarpa, S. guianensis*	Leaves	[16, 26]
Quercetin 3-*O*-β-glucopyranoside	*S. glycycarpa, S. thecaphora*	Leaves	[16, 28]
Quercetin 3-*O*-glucoside-7-*O*-rhamnoside	*S. glycycarpa, S. sarmentosa*	Leaves	[12, 17]
Quercetin 3-*O*-rhamnoside-7-*O*-glucoside	*S. glycycarpa, S. sarmentosa*	Leaves	[12, 17]
Quercetin 3-*O*-rutinoside-7-*O*-rhamnoside	*S. guianensis*	Leaves	[27]

(Table 1) cont.....

Quercetin 3,7-di-*O*-rhamnoside	*S. guianensis*	Leaves	[27]
Quercetin 3-*O*-(2”-*O*-galoyl)-pentoside	*S. glycycarpa*	Leaves	[17]
Quercetin 3-*O*-pentosyl-pentoside-7-*O*- rhamnoside	*S. guianensis*	Leaves	[27]
Quercetin 3-*O*-pentosyl-rhamnoside-7-*O*- rhamnoside	*S. guianensis*	Leaves	[27]
Quercetin 3-*O*-(6”-*O*-galoyl)-β-galacto pyranoside	*S. glycycarpa*	Leaves	[17]
***O*-Glycosylated flavonoids**			
Quercetin 3-*O*-[β-D-xylosyl-(1→2)- β-D-glucoside]	*S. glycycarpa*	Leaves	[16]
Rutin	*S. gigantotepala, S. glycycarpa, S. guianensis, S. sarmentosa, S. thecaphora*	Leaves	[12,14, 16,17,26,28]
Siparunoside	*S. brasiliensis*	Leaves	[9]
Tiliroside	*S. brasiliensis, S. glycycarpa*	Leaves	[9, 10, 16]
***C*-Glycosylated flavonoids**			
Lucenin-2	*S. guianensis*	Leaves	[27]
Vicenin-2	*S. guianensis, S. sarmentosa*	Leaves	[12, 27]
Terpenoids			
Sipaucine A, B, and C	*S. pauciflora*	Leaves	[23]
Sitosterol glycoside	*S. brasiliensis, S. guianensis*	Leaves, fruit	[9, 21]
Sitosterol	*S. brasiliensis,, S. guianensis*	Leaves, fruit	[9]
Stigmasterol	*S. brasiliensis, S. guianensis*	Leaves, stem wood	[9]
trans-Thujane-1α,7-diol 1-*O*-β-D-glycopyranoside	*S. thecaphora*	Leaves	[28]
Other Compounds			
Protocatechuic acid (Phenolic acid)	*S. glycycarpa*	Leaves	[16]
Safrole (Phenylpropanoid)	*S. guianensis*	Leaves	[30]
Dillapiole (Phenylpropanoid)	*S. guianensis*	Leaves	[30]
Pheophytin A (Pheophytin)	*S. sarmentosa*	Leaves	[12]
4-Methoxy-2-methylcinnamic acid (Cinnamic acid derivatives)	*S. sessiliflora*	Leaves	[29]
3,4-dihydroxybenzaldehyde (Phenolic aldehyde)	*S. thecaphora*	Leaves	[28]

*(syn. *S. apiosyce*).

Table 2. Chemical composition of essential oils from *Siparuna* species.

Plant Species	Chemical Compounds	Plant Part	Refs.
S. aspera	α-pinene, β-pinene, camphene, myrcene, limonene, 1,8-cineole, (*Z*)--cimene, α-terpineol, β-elemene, δ-elemene, α-cubebene, β-cubebene, α-ylangene, α-copaene, β-copaene, β-bourbomnene, cyclosativene, isolongifolene, *E*-β-caryophyllene, β-gurjunene, γ-gurjunene, α-guaiene, aristolene, *cis*-muurola-3,5-diene, α-muurolene, γ-muurolene, α-humulene, *allo*-aromadendrene, *cis*-cadina-1(6),4-diene, *trans*-cadin--1(2),4-diene, 9-*epi*-caryophyllene, bicyclogermacrene, germacrene A, germacrene B, germacrene D, β-selinene, valencene, β-himachalene, α-cadinene, γ-cadinene, δ-cadinene, α-calacoirene, spathulenol, caryophyllene oxide, viridiflorol, guaiol, β-oplopenone, 1,10-di-*epi*-cubenol, 1-*epi*-cubenol, epi- α-cadinol, α-cadinol, *epi*-α-muurolol, α-muurolol, khusinol, eudesma-4(15),7- dien-1-β-ol.	Leaves	[16]
S. echinata	α-pinene, β-pinene, β-elemene, germacrene A, germacrene B, germacrene D, α-hymulene, β-eudesmol, β-selinene, *trans*-caryophylle, camphene, sabinene, β-myrcene, limonene, *cis*-ocimene, *trans*-ocimene, perillene, caryophyllene oxide, linalool, *trans*-pinocarveol, *cis*-verbenol, nopinone, myrtenol, 6-undecanol, 2-undecanoine, 2-tridecanone, undecanoic acid.	Dried fruits	[20]
S. eggersii	α-pinene, β-pinene, β-elemene, γ-elemene, δ-elemene, camphene, α-cubebene, β-cubebene, sabinene, myrcene, limonene, α-phelandrene, β-phelandrene, *cis*-β-ocimene, *trans*-β-ocimene, linalool, elemol, α-copaene, *allo*-ocimene, *trans*-caryophyllene, α-guaiene, aromadendrene, *trans*-β-farnesene, α-humulene, δ-muurolene, β-selinene, germacrene A, germacrene B, germacrene D, germacrene-D-4-ol, bicyclogermacrene, α-farnesene, β-bourbunene, spathuletol, caryophyllene oxide, γ-cadinene, curzerenone, *epi*-α-curzerenone, α-cadinol, muurolol, sabinyl acetate, viridiflorol, decanal, 2-tridecanone.	Leaves	[21]
S. guianensis	α-pinene, β-pinene, α-limonene, D-limonene, terpineol, linalool, α-phellandrene, β-phellandrene, δ-3-carene, *p*-cymene, β-bourbunene, β-myrcene, (*E*)-β-ocimene, (*Z*)-β-ocimene, camphene, terpinolene, β-elemene, γ-elemene, δ-elemene, germacrone, germacrene A, germacrene B, germacrene D, bicyclogermacrene, curzerenone, α-bisabolol, santolina triene, α-caryophylle, β-caryophullene, *E*-caryophyllene, β-caryophyllene oxide, α-amorphene, γ-cadinene, δ-cadinene, α-copaene, β-copaene, α-cubebene, β-cubebene, curzerene, aromadendrene, humulene, humulene II epoxide, β-selinene, *trans*-calamenene, α-muurolene, γ-muurolene, cyclosativene, α-ylangen, β-ylange, valencene, β-bisabolene, α-calacorene, *cis*-sesquisabinenehydrate, α-gurjunene, β-gurjunene, γ-gurjunene, *trans*-α-bergamoptene, *Z*-β-farnesene, α-curcumene, cubebol, *epi*-cubebol, α-cadinol, *epi*-α-cadinol δ-cadinol, *T*-cadinol, ledol, spathulenol, *E*,*E*-farnesol, globulol, viridiflorol,	Leaves, stem, fruits	[9, 30 - 37]

(Table 2) cont.....

Plant Species	Chemical Compounds	Plant Part	Refs.
S. guianensis	*epi*-α-bisabolol, cubenol, 1-*epi*-cubenol, β-eudesmol, γ-eudesmol, agarospirol, siparunone, ipsdienol, elemol, guaiol, α-muurolol, selin-1--en-4-α-ol, *cis*-β-elemone, *trans*-β-elemone, 2-tridecanone, 2-undecanone, nonanol, decanol, undecanol, fatty acids.	Leaves, stem, fruits	[9, 30 - 37]
S. macrotepala	α-pinene, β-pinene, camphene, myrcene, limonene, α-cubebene, β-cubebene, cyclosativene, α-ylangene, α-copaene, β-copaene, β-bourbunene, α-cadinene, δ-cadinene, γ-cadinene, *trans*-cadina-1(2)-4-diene, β-caryophyllene, β-elemene, caryophyllene oxide, α-guayene, *cis*-muurola-3,5-diene, *trans*-muurola-3,5-diene, *cis*-muurola-4(14)-5-diene, *trans*-muurola-4(14),5-diene, humulene, *allo*-aromadendrene, α-muurolene, g-muurolene, germacrene B, germacrene D, bicuyclogermacrene, β-selinene, *E,E*,-α-farnesene, cubebol, 1-*epi*-cubenol, 1,2-di-*epi*-cubenol, globulol, viridiflorol, guaiol, α-muurolol, epi-α-muurolol, α-cadinol, *epi*-α-cadinol, spathulenol, undecanone.	Branches, leaves	[9, 16, 38]
S. schimpffii	myrcene, α-pinene, β-pinene, thujene, β-bourbunene, β-caryophyllene, α-cubebene, copaene, β-cubebene, β-elemene, δ-elemene, cyclosativene, α-guayene, α-humulene, α-ylangene, *cis*-muurola-4(14),5-diene, *cis*-muurola-3,5-diene, germacrene B, germacrene D, bicyclogermacrene, β-selinene, α-muurolene, γ-muurolene, γ-amorphene, α-cadinene, γ-cadinene, α-calcorene, nootkatone, viridiflorol, spathulenol, guaiol, 1,10-di-*epi*-cubenol, 1-*epi*-cubenol, cedrelanol, α-muurolol, tau-muurolol, α-cadinol, undecanone.	Leaves	[40]

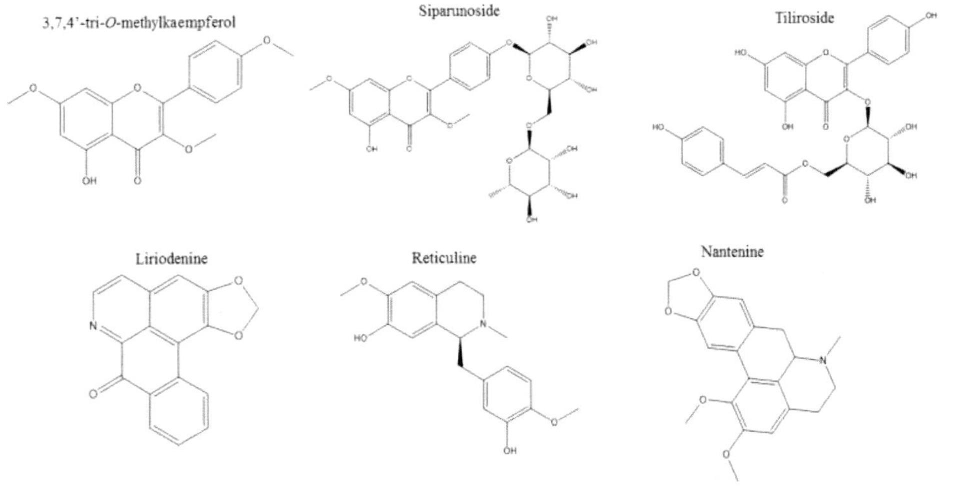

Fig. (2). Chemical structure of some flavonoids and alkaloids isolated from *Siparuna* species.

3. ANTIVIRAL POTENTIAL OF BRAZILIAN *SIPARUNA*

3.1. Antiviral Activity Against Influenza A(H1N1) Virus

Influenza, or flu, as it is usually called, is an acute viral infection of the respiratory tract caused by *Alphainfluenzavirus*, causing fever, dry cough, muscle and joint pain, headache, sore throat, and runny nose [41, 42]. There are four types of seasonal influenza viruses *Alphainfluenzavirus*, *Betainfluenzavirus*, *Deltainfluenzavirus* and *Gammainfluenzavirus* and what differs from one another are the compositions of their nuclear and matrix proteins [41 - 43]. *Alphainfluenzaviruses* and *Betainfluenzaviruses* cause seasonal epidemics of the disease being the *alpha-type* (influenzavirus A) found in mammalian species (including humans) and birds, the most significant in human morbidity and mortality [41]. Influenzavirus A subtypes (H1N1, H2N2, H3N2, H5N1) were responsible for global influenza pandemics that marked history. H1N1 was the etiological agent of the Spanish flu in 1918 with 40-50 million deaths worldwide and swine flu in 2009. H2N2 caused the Asian flu in 1957, causing more than one million deaths worldwide. In 2004, H5N1 caused avian influenza and the H3N2 virus was responsible for Hong Kong influenza in 1968 [44]. Currently, H3N2 was also responsible for influenza outbreaks that began in July 2020 in the Kingdom of Cambodia during the COVID-19 pandemic, extending to different states of Brazil, increasing the number of infection cases [45].

The *Alphainfluenzavirus* is pleomorphic (100 nm in diameter), consisting of simple tape RNA, octa-segmented, with negative polarity, coated by a nucleocapsid with helical symmetry and, externally, by a lipid envelope, where glycoproteins hemagglutinin (HA) and neuraminidase (NA) are inserted [42, 46]. NA is a therapeutic target for the development of anti-influenza drugs due to its crucial role in viral dispersion [42]. Eighteen subtypes of HA (H1 to H18) and eleven NA (N1 to N11) were identified for this type of virus and currently, subtypes A(H1N1) and A(H3N2) circulate in humans and cause seasonal epidemics [41, 42, 46].

Among the main antiviral classes available for the treatment of Influenza infections, stand the antiviral neuraminidase inhibitors (NAIs) Zanamivir (Relenza®), Oseltamivir (Tamiflu®) and Peramivir (Rapiacta®), approved by the Food and Drug Administration (FDA), which are active against influenza type *alpha*- and *beta*- [42]. NAIs bind to the active site of neuraminidase (NA), preventing the cleavage of sialic acid and consequently, the release of influenza virus into the respiratory tract, being indicated in Brazil for patients presenting severe acute respiratory syndrome [47, 48].

As stated before, natural products have been shown as sources of compounds with antiviral potential [49 - 51], as an example, we can cite Oseltamivir, which originated by semi-synthesis of shikimic acid isolated from *Illicium verum* [52]. In addition, ethanol extracts of propolis showed activity against the influenza A virus (H1N1) *in vitro* and diarylheptanoids isolated from *Alpinia officinarum* also exhibited a potential against the influenza virus *in vitro* [53].

Among the classes of secondary metabolites produced by plants, flavonoids stand out as inhibitors of the influenza virus, enabling their use as antiviral neuraminidase inhibitors [52]. Flavonoid backbones bearing glucosides, hydroxyl and methyl groups may be related to antiviral activity as well as the presence of C2=C3 double bond [54]. Flavonoids with *C*-methylation isolated from *Cleistocalyx operculatus* [52], isorhamnetin, which presents methyl group in ring B [55], (2*S*)-6,8-dimethyl-4′-metoxy-5,3′,5′-trihydroxyflavano-7-*O*-β-D-gluco-pyranoside isolated from *Matteuccia struthiopteris* rhizomes [56], are examples of flavonoids that showed activity against the Influenza H1N1 virus. Moreover, recent research showed that tiliroside from *Hibiscus mutabilis* L. inhibited four influenza A virus strains in MDCK cells with EC_{50} 3.85 to 27.81 µM and decreased the expression of cytokines/chemokines in infected cells and animal models [57]. Previous studies describe that tiliroside was isolated from the leaves of *Siparuna brasiliensis* (=*S. apiosyce*) [9, 10]. Other compounds, such as alkaloids, coumarins, gallic acid and tannins also inhibited the replication of this virus [52, 58, 59].

Recent studies by our research group evaluated the antiviral potential of 25 extracts obtained from five *Siparuna* species, *S. cristata*, *S. decipiens*, *S. glycy-carpa*, *S. reginae* and *S. sarmentosa* against influenza A(H1N1)pdm09 virus [12], showing the *n*-BuOH extracts from *S. glycycarpa* and *S. sarmentosa* as the most active, inhibiting 96.0 ± 1.3% and 89.5 ± 0.8% of influenza A(H1N1)pdm09 virus replication *in vitro* respectively, in the concentration of 100 $\mu g.mL^{-1}$ 24 h post-infection, being maintained up to 72 hpi. Among these promising extracts, alkaloids, *O*- and *C*-glycosylated flavonoids, dihydrochalcones, and a B-type procyanidin dimer could be annotated [12]. Following these first results, the *n*-BuOH extract from *S. glycycarpa* was fractionated by centrifugal partition chromatography (CPC) in descending mode, with the polar solvent system BuOH-MeOH-H_2O (9:1:10, *v/v*). Among the collected fractions, four of them showed the highest inhibition of viral replication (above 74%) at the concentration of 100 $\mu g.mL^{-1}$ after 24 hpi. Through LC-HR-MS/MS analysis of these fractions, benzylisoquinoline alkaloids were annotated in three of them, and aporphine alkaloids, *O*-glycosylated flavonoids, and dihydrochalcones in the fourth one [17].

3.2. Antiviral Activity Against SARS-CoV-2

The new severe acute respiratory syndrome coronavirus-2 (SARS-CoV-2), a kind of *Betacoronavirus*, was first identified in Wuhan city in the People's Republic of China (PRC) at the end of 2019, causing what was later declared by UN as the pandemic of COVID-19, leading to public health concerns [60, 61]. The term multiple organ dysfunction syndrome, MODS-CoV-2 was further proposed due to the high complexity of the pathophysiology of SARS-CoV-2 infection, involving not only the activation of the immune and hematologic systems but also the impairment of different organs and the potential for systemic complications [11, 62].

The act of coughing, sneezing, shouting, singing, and even talking may produce respiratory droplets in high quantities allowing the virus to be transmitted from human to human. The virus can survive on various surfaces from a few seconds to many days [60]. Although mild cold-like symptoms are often described for the disease, it may have lethal consequences following thromboembolisms, hyperinflammation and cytokine storm eventually leading to pulmonary fibrosis and multiple organ failure [63, 64].

Up to now (January 2nd, 2023), a number of 660,607,091 cases have been reported worldwide, and up to 6,690,809 fatalities have been attributed to the infection [65]. In Brazil, 36,331,601 cases were notified and 693,853 deaths from the disease were reported [66].

Vaccination programs have been successfully launched in various countries as there is an urge to immunize the entire population. Despite many advances and efforts, there is still a long delay in the supply of immunizers, especially in the most remote regions. Moreover, the duration of immunity remains yet to be studied being susceptible to novel SARS-CoV-2 strains. These facts lead to the need of exploring additional therapeutic arsenal, including those derived from medicinal plants [60].

The illness is still a health concern since outbreaks continue to resurge caused by the appearance of mutants of the virus that resist the vaccines, making it urgent need for therapeutic agents that can block SARS-CoV-2 transmission and the progression from infection to severe symptomatic illness [64].

The non-structural proteins 3-chymotrypsin-like protease (3CLpro), papain-like protease (PLpro), and RNA-dependent RNA polymerase (RdRp) and the structural spike protein (S protein), present in the SARS-CoV-2 genome, have been some of the targets for researching new drugs against this virus [11, 67]. One important feature of SARS-CoV-2 is the binding of the amino acid sequence RBD (receptor binding domain) of the Spike protein to human angiotensin-converting enzyme 2 (ACE2), used as a receptor for epithelial and endothelial cell attachment [64, 68]. So, proteases are important therapeutic targets due to their key role in the cycle of viral replication [11].

Due to this worldwide scenario, several strategies concerning the development of vaccines as well as the search for medicines (including natural medicines), monoclonal antibodies, interferon therapies and peptides, have been the focus of different research groups for fighting the new coronavirus [11]. Natural products could be a valuable source of new lead compounds or drugs for the handling of COVID-19 disease, given that they can act on multi targets and through different mechanisms [64, 69].

Current literature reports *ca.* 130 natural products with antiviral potential, distributed in different classes such as alkaloids, flavonoids, terpenoids, and others. Among them, 94 metabolites demonstrated bioactivity against coronaviruses where most of them were flavonoid derivatives [70].

If we consider the different targets in the "battle fronts" against coronavirus it is possible to observe several natural products acting as inhibitors of either the S protein or enzymes (proteases and RNA polymerases) which are key enzymes in viral replication such as 3CLpro, PLpro, helicase, and RdRp. Boozari and co-workers [71], in a recent review on natural products for COVID-19 prevention and treatment mentioned emodin (an anthraquinone derivative) and baicalin (a glycosylated flavonoid) as inhibitors of the S protein, as well as iguesterin (a quinone-methide triterpene) as an inhibitor of 3CLpro. Another flavonoid, the biflavone sotetsuflavone is cited as an inhibitor of RdRp and the abietane diterpenequimone cryptotanshinone, an inhibitor of PLpro. The group also mentions that different types of terpenoids have promising effects as inhibitors of viral replication and that some alkaloids such as homoharringtonine, lycorine, and emetine have strong anti-coronavirus effects [71].

From all cited classes of natural products, flavonoids are potential candidates to fight the coronavirus by interfering with its lifecycle as they have been shown to exhibit inhibitory activity against pivotal viral targets, required to facilitate their entry and replication, including M^{pro}, RBD of the S protein, RdRp, in addition to the human ACE-2 receptor and TMPRSS2 (an endothelial cell surface protein that is involved in the viral entry and spread of coronaviruses including SARS-CoV-2). This class of compounds has safe administration with a lack of systemic toxicity. Quercetin and luteolin, two flavonoid aglycones, stand out as promising compounds as they exhibit multi-target activity against SARS-CoV-2. One reason could be related to the ability of flavonoids to work synergistically even with other drugs as their functional groups can interact with different cellular targets intercepting multiple pathways [72, 73].

Methylated flavonoids isolated by our group from the dichloromethane extract of leaves of *Siparuna cristata* using high-speed countercurrent chromatography (HSCCC) with the solvent system hexane-ethyl acetate-methanol-water (1:1:1:1, *v/v*): 3,3′,4′-tri-*O*-methyl-quercetin, 3,7,3′,4′-tetra-*O*-methyl-quercetin (retusin), and 3,7-di-*O*-methyl-kaempferol (kumatakenin) were investigated for their inhibitory effect against SARS-CoV-2 viral replication. The flavonoids retusin and kumatakenin (Fig. **3**) isolated by this technique were able to inhibit viral replication of SARS-CoV-2 with EC_{50} values of 0.4 ± 0.05 (Vero E6) and 0.6 ± 0.06 (Calu-3) for retusin, and EC_{50} 10 ± 0.7 (Vero E6) and 0.3 ± 0.02 (Calu-3) for kumatakenin. These two compounds also showed a higher selectivity index than the controls lopinavir/ritonavir and chloroquine [11].

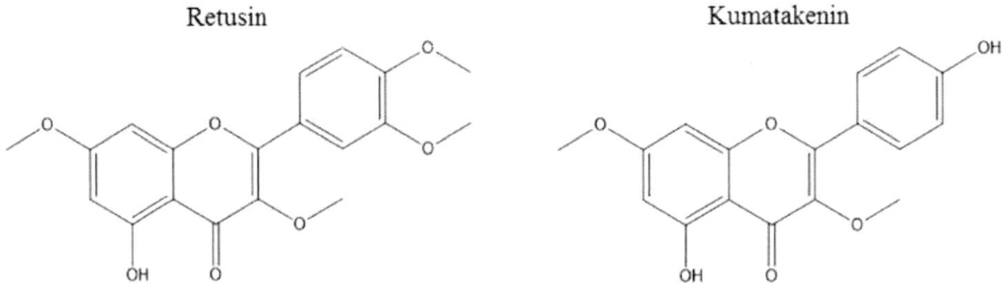

Fig. (3). Structures of the flavonoids inhibiting SARS-CoV-2 replication.

Furthermore, *in-silico* results [11] demonstrated the potential interaction between the two flavonoids and key residues of COVID-19 3CLpro as well as PLpro, in a similar way to that of the screened potential inhibitors against COVID-19. Even though all three tested flavonoids showed good results in the assays, retusin presented the best results both in the antiviral replication assay and the molecular docking based on the hydrogen-bonding distance between selected amino acid residues of the catalytic site from 3CLpro and PLpro SARS-CoV-2 proteases. The results of this study highlight the possible application of methylated flavonoids, for example retusin, as an antiviral or adjuvant therapy in the treatment of COVID-19.

Other *in silico* studies analyzed the interaction of terpenes from the essential oil of *Siparuna guianensis* with SARS-CoV-2 proteins and human angiotensin-converting enzyme 2 (hACE2) by molecular docking and AutoDock Vina software [74]. The authors describe that the best-docked interaction corresponded to the sesquiterpenes identified in the essential oil: γ-eudesmol with hACE2, SARS-CoV-2 main protease, SARS-CoV-2 Nsp15/NendoU, and SARS-CoV RdRp; spathulenol and γ-eudesmol with SARS-CoV RdRp; and *t*-muurolol with Spike S macromolecules. As for the main result, γ-eudesmol showed the best interaction energy with various macromolecules involved in the SARS-CoV-2 infection [74]. Based on these results, the authors suggest that the essential oil of *S. guianensis* should be further investigated by *in vitro* and *in vivo* studies, being a promising herbal therapeutic adjuvant against SARS-CoV-2 infections.

CONCLUSION

The anti-influenza A(H1N1)pdm09 and anti-SARS-CoV-2 activity of *Siparuna* species show their potential for bioprospecting antiviral agents. The data described so far in the literature corroborate the use of plants of this genus in Brazilian folk medicine for the treatment and prophylaxis of respiratory diseases. The promising results stimulate the continuation of studies to investigate the chemical composition of their extracts and fractions, as well as the search for compounds that may be related to these bioactivities for the development of and for obtaining new antivirals of natural origin, active against pathogens of great clinical importance.

REFERENCES

[1] Lin LT, Hsu WC, Lin CC. Antiviral natural products and herbal medicines. J Tradit Complement Med 2014; 4(1): 24-35.
[http://dx.doi.org/10.4103/2225-4110.124335] [PMID: 24872930]

[2] Musarra-Pizzo M, Pennisi R, Ben-Amor I, Mandalari G, Sciortino MT. Antiviral activity exerted by natural products against human viroses. Viruses 2021; 13(5): 828.
[http://dx.doi.org/10.3390/v13050828] [PMID: 34064347]

[3] Kitazato K, Wang Y, Kobayashi N. Viral infectious disease and natural products with antiviral activity. Drug Discov Ther 2007; 1(1): 14-22.
[PMID: 22504360]

[4] Yuan H, Ma Q, Ye L, Piao G. The traditional medicine and modern medicine from natural products. Molecules 2016; 21(5): 559.
[http://dx.doi.org/10.3390/molecules21050559] [PMID: 27136524]

[5] Badshah SL, Faisal S, Muhammad A, Poulson BG, Emwas AH, Jaremko M. Antiviral activities of flavonoids. Biomed Pharmacother 2021; 140: 111596.
[http://dx.doi.org/10.1016/j.biopha.2021.111596] [PMID: 34126315]

[6] Renner SS, Schwarzbach AE, Lohmann L. Phylogenetic position and floral function of siparuna *(Siparunaceae:Laurales)*. Int J Plant Sci 1997; 158(S6): S89-98.
[http://dx.doi.org/10.1086/297509]

[7] Renner SS, Hausner G. Siparunaceae in: Flora neotropica. monograph 95. New York Botanical Garden 2005; 256: 1016.

[8] Silva IF, Oliveira FF, Oliveira ADO. ARA. Siparuna Aublet genus (Siparunaceae): From folk medicine to chemical composition and biological activity. Trends Phytochem 2021; 5: 168-89.
[http://dx.doi.org/10.30495/tpr.2021.1934361.1211]

[9] Leitão GG, Simas NK, Soares SSV, *et al.* Chemistry and pharmacology of monimiaceae: A special focus on *Siparuna* and *mollinedia.* J Ethnopharmacol 1999; 65(2): 87-102. [http://dx.doi.org/10.1016/S0378-8741(98)00233-5] [PMID: 10465659]

[10] Leitão GG, Soares SSV, Brito M, Delle Monache F, de Barros T. Kaempferol glycosides from siparuna apiosyce. Phytochemistry 2000; 55(6): 679-82. [http://dx.doi.org/10.1016/S0031-9422(00)00222-3] [PMID: 11130680]

[11] Leal CM, Leitão SG, Sausset R, *et al.* Flavonoids from *Siparuna cristata* as potential inhibitors of SARS-CoV-2 replication. Rev Bras Farmacogn 2021; 31(5): 658-66. [http://dx.doi.org/10.1007/s43450-021-00162-5] [PMID: 34305198]

[12] Leal CM, Simas RC, Miranda M, *et al.* Amazonian *Siparuna* extracts as potential anti-influenza agents: Metabolic fingerprinting. J Ethnopharmacol 2021; 270: 113788. [http://dx.doi.org/10.1016/j.jep.2021.113788] [PMID: 33429033]

[13] Moura AS, Machado FS, Mariano RF, Trotta RR, Fontes MAL. Fruit consuption and dispersion to siparuna guianensis *(Siparunaceae)* by Guerlinguetus *(ingrami)* brasiliensis *(Mammalia:Rodentia)* in siutheastern brazil. Nature Onl 2017; 15: 014-7.

[14] Torres Castañeda HG, Colmenares Dulcey AJ, Isaza Martínez JH. Flavonoid glycosides from *Siparuna gigantotepala* leaves and their antioxidant activity. Chem Pharm Bull 2016; 64(5): 502-6. [http://dx.doi.org/10.1248/cpb.c15-00788] [PMID: 27150483]

[15] Facundo VA, Azevedo MS, Rodrigues RV, *et al.* Chemical constituents from three medicinal plants: *Piper renitens, Siparuna guianensis* and *Alternanthera brasiliana.* Rev Bras Farmacogn 2012; 22(5): 1134-9. [http://dx.doi.org/10.1590/S0102-695X2012005000040]

[16] Costa FN, Garrard I, da Silva AJR, Leitão GG. Changes in the mobile phase composition on a stepwise counter-current chromatography elution for the isolation of flavonoids from *Siparuna glycycarpa.* J Sep Sci 2013; 36(14): 2253-9. [http://dx.doi.org/10.1002/jssc.201201054] [PMID: 23686916]

[17] Leal CM, Leitão SG, de Mello LLO, *et al.* Bioassay-guided fractionation of *Siparuna glycycarpa n*-butanol extract with inhibitory activity against influenza A(H1N1)pdm09 virus by centrifugal partition chromatography (CPC). Molecules 2022; 27(2): 399. [http://dx.doi.org/10.3390/molecules27020399] [PMID: 35056716]

[18] Marti G, Eparvier V, Morleo B, *et al.* Natural aristolactams and aporphine alkaloids as inhibitors of CDK1/cyclin B and DYRK1A. Molecules 2013; 18(3): 3018-27. [http://dx.doi.org/10.3390/molecules18033018] [PMID: 23467012]

[19] López DHP. Evaluation of the antibacterial activity of the alkaloids from the leaves of Siparuna sessiliflora. Faculty of chemistry Bogotá. Pontifical Javeriana University 2011; pp. 65-72.

[20] Braz Fo R, Gabriel SJ, Gomes CMR, Gottlieb OR, Bichara MDGA, Maia JGS. Oxoaporphine alkaloids from *Fusea longifolia* and *Siparuna guianensis.* Phytochemistry 1976; 15(7): 1187-8. [http://dx.doi.org/10.1016/0031-9422(76)85135-7]

[21] Simas NK, Ferrari SF, Pereira SN, Leitão GG. Chemical ecological characteristics of herbivory of Siparuna guianensis seeds by buffy-headed marmosets (Callithrix flaviceps) in the atlantic forest of southeastern brazil. J Chem Ecol 2001; 27(1): 93-107. [http://dx.doi.org/10.1023/A:1005672017673] [PMID: 11382070]

[22] Fischer DCH, Gonçalves MI, Oliveira F, Alvarenga MA. Phytochemical communication. Fitot 1999; 70: 322.

[23] Jenett-Siems K, Kraft C, Siems K, *et al.* Sipaucins A–C, sesquiterpenoids from *Siparuna pauciflora.* Phytochemistry 2003; 63(4): 377-81. [http://dx.doi.org/10.1016/S0031-9422(03)00098-0] [PMID: 12770583]

[24] Gerard RV, MacLean DB, Antonio TM. Examination of three *Siparuna* species for alkaloid content. Phytochemistry 1986; 25(9): 2155-6.
[http://dx.doi.org/10.1016/0031-9422(86)80080-2]

[25] Chiu SYC, Dobberstein RH, Fong HHS, Farnsworth NR. Oxoaporphine alkaloids from *Siparuna gilgiana.* J Nat Prod 1982; 45(2): 229-30.
[http://dx.doi.org/10.1021/np50020a024]

[26] Guimarães Leitão G, Santos El-Adji S, de Melo WAL, Guimarães Leitão S, Brown L. Separation of free and glycosylated flavonoids from *Siparuna guianensis* by gradient and isocratic CCC. J Liq Chromatogr Relat Technol 2005; 28(12-13): 2041-51.
[http://dx.doi.org/10.1081/JLC-200063669]

[27] Negri G, Santi D, Tabach R. Chemical composition of hydroethanolic extracts from *Siparuna guianensis*, medicinal plant used as anxiolytics in Amazon region. Rev Bras Farmacogn 2012; 22(5): 1024-34.
[http://dx.doi.org/10.1590/S0102-695X2012005000034]

[28] Vera Saltos MB, Naranjo Puente BF, Malafronte N, Braca A. A new monoterpene glycoside from *Siparuna thecaphora*. Nat Prod Res 2014; 28(1): 57-60.
[http://dx.doi.org/10.1080/14786419.2013.843179] [PMID: 24087860]

[29] González GFP, Archila EG. Anti-bacterial action of extracts and fractions from *Siparuna sessiliflor*a Kunth A. DC. (limoncillo). Rev Cuba Plantas Med 2012; 17: 65. Corpus ID: 101105295.

[30] Antonio TM, Waller GR, Mussinan CJ. Composition of essential oil from the leaves of *Siparuna guianensis* (Monimiaceae). Chem Ind 1984; 14: 514.

[31] Santana de Oliveira M, da Cruz JN, Almeida da Costa W, *et al.* Chemical composition, antimicrobial properties of *Siparuna guianensis* essential oil and a molecular docking and dynamics molecular study of its major chemical constituent. Molecules 2020; 25(17): 3852.
[http://dx.doi.org/10.3390/molecules25173852] [PMID: 32854178]

[32] Zoghbi MGB, Andrade EHA, Santos AS, Silva MHL, Maia JGS. Essential oils of *Siparuna guianensis* Aubl. J Essent Oil Res 1998; 10(5): 543-6.
[http://dx.doi.org/10.1080/10412905.1998.9700966]

[33] Andrade M, das Graças Cardoso M, de Andrade J, *et al.* Chemical composition and antioxidant activity of essential oils from *Cinnamodendron dinisii* Schwacke and *Siparuna guianensis* Aublet. Antioxidants 2013; 2(4): 384-97.
[http://dx.doi.org/10.3390/antiox2040384] [PMID: 26784471]

[34] Aguiar RWS, dos Santos SF, da Silva Morgado F, *et al.* Insecticidal and repellent activity of *Siparuna guianensis* Aubl. (Negramina) against *Aedes aegypti* and *Culex quinquefasciatus.* PLoS One 2015; 10(2): e0116765.
[http://dx.doi.org/10.1371/journal.pone.0116765] [PMID: 25646797]

[35] Melo DC, Miranda MLD, Júnior WGF, *et al.* Anticariogenic and antimycobacterial activities of the essential oil of *Siparuna guianensis* Aublet (Siparunaceae). Orbital: The Electronic. J Chem 2017; 9: 55.
[http://dx.doi.org/10.17807/orbital.v0i0.930]

[36] Lourenço AM, Haddi K, Ribeiro BM, *et al.* Essential oil of *Siparuna guianensis* as an alternative tool for improved lepidopteran control and resistance management practices. Sci Rep 2018; 8(1): 7215.
[http://dx.doi.org/10.1038/s41598-018-25721-0] [PMID: 29740112]

[37] Ferreira TP, Oliveira EE, Tschoeke PH, Pinheiro RG, Maia AMS, Aguiar RWS. Potential use of negramina (*Siparuna guianensis* Aubl.) essential oil to control wax moths and its selectivity in relation to honey bees. Ind Crops Prod 2017; 109: 151-7.
[http://dx.doi.org/10.1016/j.indcrop.2017.08.023]

[38] El-Seedi H, Ghia F, Torssell KBG. Cadinane sesquiterpenes from *Siparuna macrotepala.*

Phytochemistry 1994; 35(6): 1495-7. [http://dx.doi.org/10.1016/S0031-9422(00)86883-1]

[39] Rivera PFN, Guerrini A, Tsamaraint EA. Chemical composition of leaf essential oil of *Siparuna schimpffii* Diels (limoncillo). Rev Cuba Plantas Med 2014; 19: 128.

[40] Morocho V, Hidalgo-Tapia M, Delgado-Loyola I, Cartuche L, Cumbicus N, Valarezo E. Chemical composition and biological activity of essential oil from leaves and fruits of Limoncilo (Siparuna muricata (Ruiz & Pav.) A. DC.). Antibiotics 2023; 12(1): 82. [http://dx.doi.org/10.3390/antibiotics12010082] [PMID: 36671283]

[41] World Health Organization (WHO). Influenza. 2018. Available From: http://www.who.int/mediacentre/factsheets/fs211/en/ (Accessed on 2 Jan 2023)

[42] Ai W, Zhang J, Zalloum WA, *et al.* Discovery of novel *Dual-site* binding oseltamivir derivatives as potent influenza virus neuraminidase inhibitors. Eur J Med Chem 2020; 191: 112147. [http://dx.doi.org/10.1016/j.ejmech.2020.112147] [PMID: 32092589]

[43] international committee on taxonomy of viruses (ICTV). 2021. Available From: https://talk.ictvonline.org/ictv-reports/ictv_9th_report/negative-sense-rna-viruses-2011/w/negrna_viruses/209/orthomyxoviridae (Accessed on 2 May 2022).

[44] Setzer WN. Essential oils as complementary and alternative medicines for the treatment of influenza. Amer J Essential Oils Nat Prod 2016; 4: 16. Corpus ID: 54815123.

[45] Sovann LY, Sar B, Kab V, *et al.* An influenza A (H3N2) virus outbreak in the Kingdom of Cambodia during the COVID-19 pandemic of 2020. Int J Infect Dis 2021; 103: 352-7. [http://dx.doi.org/10.1016/j.ijid.2020.11.178] [PMID: 33249287]

[46] de Vries E, Du W, Guo H, de Haan CAM. Influenza A virus hemagglutinin-neuraminidase-receptor balance: Preserving virus motility. Trends Microbiol 2020; 28(1): 57-67. [http://dx.doi.org/10.1016/j.tim.2019.08.010] [PMID: 31629602]

[47] Das K, Aramini JM, Ma LC, Krug RM, Arnold E. Structures of influenza A proteins and insights into antiviral drug targets. Nat Struct Mol Biol 2010; 17(5): 530-8. [http://dx.doi.org/10.1038/nsmb.1779] [PMID: 20383144]

[48] Wang P, Zhang JZH. Selective binding of antiinfluenza drugs and their analogues to 'open' and 'closed' conformations of H5N1 neuraminidase. J Phys Chem B 2010; 114(40): 12958-64. [http://dx.doi.org/10.1021/jp1030224] [PMID: 20860351]

[49] Denaro M, Smeriglio A, Barreca D, *et al.* Antiviral activity of plants and their isolated bioactive compounds: An update. Phytother Res 2020; 34(4): 742-68. [http://dx.doi.org/10.1002/ptr.6575] [PMID: 31858645]

[50] Ben-Shabat S, Yarmolinsky L, Porat D, Dahan A. Antiviral effect of phytochemicals from medicinal plants: Applications and drug delivery strategies. Drug Deliv Transl Res 2020; 10(2): 354-67. [http://dx.doi.org/10.1007/s13346-019-00691-6] [PMID: 31788762]

[51] Newman DJ, Cragg GM. Natural products as sources of new drugs over the nearly four decades from 01/1981 to 09/2019. J Nat Prod 2020; 83(3): 770-803. [http://dx.doi.org/10.1021/acs.jnatprod.9b01285] [PMID: 32162523]

[52] Grienke U, Schmidtke M, von Grafenstein S, Kirchmair J, Liedl KR, Rollinger JM. Influenza neuraminidase: A druggable target for natural products. Nat Prod Rep 2012; 29(1): 11-36. [http://dx.doi.org/10.1039/C1NP00053E] [PMID: 22025274]

[53] Kurokawa M, Shimizu T, Watanabe W, Shiraki K. Development of New Antiviral Agents from Natural Products. Int J Antimicrob 2010; 2(2): 49-57. [http://dx.doi.org/10.2174/1876518101002020049]

[54] Wang T, Li Q, Bi K. Bioactive flavonoids in medicinal plants: Structure, activity and biological fate. Asian J Pharm Sci 2018; 13(1): 12-23.

[http://dx.doi.org/10.1016/j.ajps.2017.08.004] [PMID: 32104374]

[55] Dayem AA, Choi HY, Kim YB, Cho SG. Antiviral effect of methylated flavonol isorhamnetin against influenza. PLoS One 2015; 10(3): e0121610.
[http://dx.doi.org/10.1371/journal.pone.0121610] [PMID: 25806943]

[56] Li B, Ni Y, Zhu LJ, *et al.* Flavonoids from *Matteuccia struthiopteris* and Their Anti-influenza Virus (H1N1) Activity. J Nat Prod 2015; 78(5): 987-95.
[http://dx.doi.org/10.1021/np500879t] [PMID: 25927664]

[57] Xiao M, Zhang T, Cao F, *et al.* Anti-influenza properties of tiliroside isolated from hibiscus mutabilis L. J Ethno 2023; 303: 115918.
[http://dx.doi.org/10.1016/j.jep.2022.115918]

[58] Theisen LL, Erdelmeier CAJ, Spoden GA, *et al.* Tannins from *Hamamelis virginiana* bark extract: Characterization and improvement of the antiviral efficacy against influenza A virus and human papillomavirus. PLoS One 2014; 9(1): e88062.
[http://dx.doi.org/10.1371/journal.pone.0088062] [PMID: 24498245]

[59] Moradi MT, Karimi A, Lorigooini Z. Alkaloids as the natural anti-influenza virus agents: A systematic review. Toxin Rev 2017; 1.
[http://dx.doi.org/10.1080/15569543.2017.1323338]

[60] Singla RK, He X, Chopra H, *et al.* Natural products for the prevention and control of the COVID-19 Pandemic: Sustainable bioresources. Front Pharmacol 2021; 12: 758159.
[http://dx.doi.org/10.3389/fphar.2021.758159] [PMID: 34925017]

[61] Khazeei Tabari MA, Iranpanah A, Bahramsoltani R, Rahimi R. Flavonoids as promising antiviral agentes against SARS-Cov-2 infection: A mechanistic review. Molecules 2021; 26(13): 3900.
[http://dx.doi.org/10.3390/molecules26133900]

[62] Antonio AS, Wiedemann LSM, Veiga-Júnior VF. Natural products' role against COVID-19. RSC Advances 2020; 10(39): 23379-93.
[http://dx.doi.org/10.1039/D0RA03774E] [PMID: 35693131]

[63] Santana FPR, Thevenard F, Gomes KS, *et al.* New perspectives on natural flavonoids on COVID-1--induced lung injuries. Phytother Res 2021; 35(9): 4988-5006.
[http://dx.doi.org/10.1002/ptr.7131] [PMID: 33928690]

[64] Isidoro C, Chiung-Fang Chang A, Sheen LY. Natural products as a source of novel drugs for treating SARS-CoV2 infection. J Tradit Complement Med 2022; 12(1): 1-5.
[http://dx.doi.org/10.1016/j.jtcme.2022.02.001] [PMID: 35155135]

[65] World Health Organization. Coronavirus disease. 2019. Available From: https://www.who.int/emergencies/diseases/novel-coronavirus-2019 (Accessed on 2 Jan 2023).

[66] Johns Hopkins University. COVID-19 data repository by the center for systems science and engineering (JHU CSSE). Available From: https://coronavirus.jhu.edu/region/brazil (Accessed on 2 Jan 2023).

[67] da Silva FMA, da Silva KPA, de Oliveira LPM, *et al.* Flavonoid glycosides and their putative human metabolites as potential inhibitors of the SARS-CoV-2 main protease (Mpro) and RNA-dependent RNA polymerase (RdRp). Mem Inst Oswaldo Cruz 2020; 115: e200207.
[http://dx.doi.org/10.1590/0074-02760200207] [PMID: 33027419]

[68] Chakravarti R, Singh R, Ghosh A, *et al.* A review on potential of natural products in the management of COVID-19. RSC Advances 2021; 11(27): 16711-35.
[http://dx.doi.org/10.1039/D1RA00644D] [PMID: 35479175]

[69] Chauhan DS, Yadav S, Quraishi MA. Natural products as environmentally safe and green approach to combat Covid-19. Curr Opin Green Sustain Chem 2021; 4: 100114.
[http://dx.doi.org/10.1016/j.crgsc.2021.100114]

[70] Omrani M, Keshavarz M, Nejad Ebrahimi S, *et al.* Potential natural products against respiratory viruses: A perspective to develop anti-COVID-19 medicines. Front Pharmacol 2021; 11: 586993. [http://dx.doi.org/10.3389/fphar.2020.586993] [PMID: 33679384]

[71] Boozari M, Hosseinzadeh H. Natural products for COVID-19 prevention and treatment regarding to previous coronavirus infections and novel studies. Phytother Res 2021; 35(2): 864-76. [http://dx.doi.org/10.1002/ptr.6873] [PMID: 32985017]

[72] Kaul R, Paul P, Kumar S, Büsselberg D, Dwivedi VD, Chaari A. Promising antiviral activities of natural flavonoids against SARS-CoV-2 Targets: Systematic review. Int J Mol Sci 2021; 22(20): 11069. [http://dx.doi.org/10.3390/ijms222011069] [PMID: 34681727]

[73] Alzaabi MM, Hamdy R, Ashmawy NS, *et al.* Flavonoids are promising safe therapy against COVID-19. Phytochem Rev 2022; 21(1): 291-312. [http://dx.doi.org/10.1007/s11101-021-09759-z] [PMID: 34054380]

[74] Costa R, Martins R, de Lima G, *et al.* Molecular docking *in silico* analysis of Brazilian essential oils against host targets and SARS-CoV-2 proteins. J Braz Chem Soc 2022; 10: 1219. [http://dx.doi.org/10.21577/0103-5053.20220043]

CHAPTER 2

Antimicrobial and Antifungal Potential of Indian Spices

Jalpa Sanandia[1], Mousmi Patel[1] and Nasir Vadia[2,*]

[1] *Department of Pharmaceutical Sciences, Saurashtra University, Rajkot, Gujarat, India*

[2] *Department of Pharmaceutical Sciences, Faculty of Health Sciences, Marwadi University, Rajkot, Gujarat, India*

Abstract: Infectious diseases caused by pathogens and food poisoning induced by spoilage bacteria pose a global hazard to human health. Microbial resistance has harmed the efficacy of various antimicrobial drugs, which are now used to extend the shelf life, raise the safety of food products in the food business, and suppress disease-causing germs in medicine. As a result, new antimicrobial agents that can overcome resistance must be developed. Many spices, including clove, oregano, thyme, cinnamon, and cumin, were found to have significant antibacterial and antifungal activity against food spoilage bacteria like *Bacillus subtilis* and *Pseudomonas fluorescens*, pathogens like *Staphylococcus aureus* and *Vibrio parahaemolyticus*, harmful fungi like *Aspergillus flavus*, and even antibiotic-resistant microorganisms like methicillin. In addition to their flavor and aroma features, many spices and herbs used today are recognized for their antimicrobial and therapeutic properties. Plant extracts from cinnamon, clove, garlic, mustard, onion, and oregano were sensitive to most foodborne bacterial pathogens studied. The essential oil portion of spices and herbs contains many antibacterial chemicals. Antimicrobial compounds in spices were more responsive to Gram-positive bacteria than those in spices were to Gram-negative bacteria. The degree of sensitivity differed depending on the strain and climatic variables. Spices that stimulate acid generation in starting cultures can have a direct effect on the rate of fermentation. Spices contain antimicrobial compounds such as phenols, alcohols, aldehydes, ketones, ethers, and hydrocarbons. In the current chapter, Indian spices and their key antimicrobial components are explored for their antibacterial activity and ways of action.

Keywords: Antimicrobial, Indian spices, Inhibition of biofilm formation, Inhibition of the bacterial enzyme, Inhibition of DNA-RNA synthesis, Mechanism of action, Receptor modifier, Suppression of cell walls.

* **Corresponding author Nasir Vadia:** Department of Pharmaceutical Sciences, Faculty of Health Sciences, Marwadi University, Rajkot, Gujarat, India; E-mail: nasirvadia@rediff.com

1. INTRODUCTION

Spice history is the history of humanity and empires that rose and fell through the commerce of exotic spices from faraway locations and transformed our society's basic foundations in an intoxicating way. The spices trade of cinnamon and black pepper developed in South Asia and the Middle East by at least 2000 BC. The Egyptians utilized mummification plants and helped promote global trade in their thirst for exotic spices and herbs. The word "spice" is the old French word "spice" that has become "epice" and originates from the Latin root spec, which means the noun "appearance." In China, Korea, and India, by 1000 BCE, herbal medical systems could be identified. Spice is the main substance used for flavoring, coloring, or preserving foodstuff. Spices differ from the herbs used for flavoring or as garnishes, which are the plants' leaves, blossoms, or stems. Spices may sometimes made into a powder for ease of use. Spices are vital in numerous places, from the culinary and medical uses of homes. Each country produces some spice, as India is blessed with various climates. It is hardly surprising that spices are widely used to cook in India. Spices are considered particularly useful not just in India but also in certain other countries. Spices are obtained from all parts of the plant, like root, flower, flower bud, bark, leaves, stem, fruits, seed, *etc*., but herbs are considered to be obtained only from non-woody materials. There are 80 different varieties of spices grown worldwide, and roughly 50 of them are grown in India, making it a major producer of spices. Many medical enterprises, including those in the fields of cosmetics, pharmaceuticals, and aromatic fragrances, rely on spices [1]. Besides providing color and taste, spices offer endless health benefits. Spices safeguard the population's health against acute, chronic, and non-communicable diseases. The favorable benefits to human health have been thoroughly examined in numerous nations [2]. But until recently, in the Western world, the interest in spices has increased [3, 4]. Most of the positive health effects of herbs and spices towards preventing or ameliorating chronic diseases such as cancer, cardiovascular disease, arthritis, and neurodegeneration appear to be mediated through the direct action of their constituent phytochemicals (particularly polyphenols or polyphenol breakdown products) targeting specific receptors or enzymes involved in various anti-inflammatory pathways or immune responses [2]. In India, the traditional medicine -Ayurveda- places a strong stress on diet and the prevention of disease. Turmeric for jaundice, basil for heart protection, mace for stomach infections, cinnamon for circulation, and ginger, the global medicine, for nausea and indigestion are some examples of how plants and spices are used in ayurveda for health benefits. Trade between ancient Rome, China, and India, known as the "house of spices," dates back centuries. Indian spices are the most well-liked in the world today because of their exquisite flavor, aroma, and medicinal properties. The largest domestic spice market in the world is one that India contributes to. In India, where they have historically been grown on small farms, spices have lately begun to emphasize organic farming. India is the world's greatest spicy producer, user, and exporter; the country produces around 75 of the 109 kinds classified by the ISO and accounts for half of the worldwide spice trafficking. A "Masala Dabba" is one of the necessities in an Indian kitchen. The cups (usually 5 or 7) are normally small, with spices used in everyday cookery. Whether it is a soupy South Indian Rasam, Gujarati Dhokla snack, Bengal Mishti Doi sumptuously serves desserts, or Kashmiri Kahwa traditional tea, spices are common in diverse areas around the country. As opposed to other farm goods, spices are often pricey. Indian spices are quite popular worldwide. In June 2020, spice exports grew 23 percent compared with that of the same month last year. At a value of around 37 billion Indian Rupees, the United States was the top importer of Indian spices. India imports certain spices, such as Asefotieda or Hing, even as one of the largest spices suppliers. Hing has been introduced from neighboring nations, such as Afghanistan, Iran, and Uzbekistan, as the main component in traditional kitchens. Recently, India began to grow this spice, which will be another feather in the country's cape if it succeeds. In the financial year 2019, a total of US$ 2.80 billion was exported from the country, 1.10 million tonnes of pure spices and spice products, whereas in financial year 18, worth US$ 2.78 billion, represented a growth of 7% in volume. The top 10 Indian spice importing companies in the 19th century were the United States, China, Vietnam, Hong Kong, Bangladesh, Thailand, the United Kingdom, the United States, Malaysia, and Sri Lanka. During the financial year 2019, Chilies, Mint products, Pickles and Oleoresins, Curcumin, pepper, Cardamom-Pulver, other spices like Tamarind and Asafoetida, and Cassia and Garlic were the top 10 exported spices and spice products. India's export of chili during the financial year 2019 amounted to 468,500, 180,300 tonnes of cumin export, 133,600 tonnes of turmeric export, and 860 tonnes of cardamom. The overall export of spices for April 2020 was 3,55 billion dollars and 348,32 million dollars in February 2021. Ginger exports showed the biggest growth in the financial year 2020 (through December 2019), at 19.410 tonnes (47 percent), followed by cardamom at 1.060 tonnes (31 percent) and cumin at 7.350 tonnes (14 percent).

Indian cuisine uses a lot of these herbs and spices to add flavor, and large amounts can be eaten in a single dinner. These herbs and spices may also offer good antioxidants, vitamins, and minerals, including iron and calcium. An adult in India is thought to be able to consume up to 4 g of turmeric per day, which could provide 80–200 milligrams of the bioactive compound curcumin per day. According to reports, some Indians consume up to 50 g of garlic per week [5]. Some research shows that traditional food (containing Asian spices) is important to the body and helps boost immunity. Bay leaf is derived from a shrub (Laurel). It is frequently used as a spice in the Mediterranean lands and is considered a traditional medicine for treating several diseases [3]. Most Indian kitchen herbs and spices mainly contain essential oils. These essential oils are found to be active against a wide variety of viruses, such as influenza virus, human herpesviruses, human immunodeficiency virus, yellow fever virus, and avian influenza [6]. The rise of the COVID-19 pandemic has unsurprisingly led to a surge in the adoption of conventional remedies aimed at bolstering immunity [7]. A survey conducted among 531 individuals across various countries during this pandemic revealed that 71.8% of respondents rely on kadha to combat the infection and enhance their immune system. Moreover, a significant majority (86.1%) of participants believe that kadha has no adverse effects, while 13.9% hold the opposite view. Impressively, a staggering 93.6% of those surveyed are convinced that spices not only aid in combating COVID-19 and other viral infections but also play a role in boosting overall immunity. Spices and herbs are widely recognized for their various health-enhancing properties, such as being rich in antioxidants, anti-inflammatory, and possessing anti-tumorigenic and anticarcinogenic qualities. They also demonstrate glycaemic and cholesterol-lowering effects and cognitive and humoral benefits. Over the past decade, researchers have uncovered numerous health advantages associated with the presence of sulfide-containing chemicals, tannins, alkaloids, phenolic diterpenes, and essential vitamins, notably flavonoids and polyphenols, in these natural ingredients. Regular consumption of spicy meals has been notably linked to reduced risks of mortality from cancer, ischemic heart disease, and respiratory system ailments. Nevertheless, the true significance of spices and herbs in promoting overall health remains uncertain, particularly concerning their potential to protect against the development of chronic, non-communicable diseases.

Indian spices possess a diverse range of physiological and pharmacological properties that contribute to promoting and protecting health against various chronic ailments. Fig. (**1**) highlights some essential therapeutic activities associated with these spices. Saffron, curcumin, the pepper family, zingiber, and cinnamon are among the identified spices known for their potential in treating conditions such as hypercholesterolemia, cardiovascular disease, obesity, inflammation/metabolic disorders, diabetes, and Alzheimer's disease. Indian spices, particularly cinnamon and curcumin, have gained significance as biotherapies in both industrialized and developing nations. They play a crucial role in modulating the immune system and serving as antimicrobial agents. Incorporating cinnamon and curcumin into nutrition interventions has shown promise in addressing chronic diseases worldwide. Moreover, they are employed in medication and hormone biotherapy, with specific doses of these spices being used. In the case of diabetes therapeutics, cinnamon and curcumin have proven beneficial in managing plasma hyperglycemia and regulating insulin dosage and frequency. Cinnamon, in particular, has demonstrated its ability to control insulin levels and counteract hyperglycemia-induced mitochondrial apoptosis.

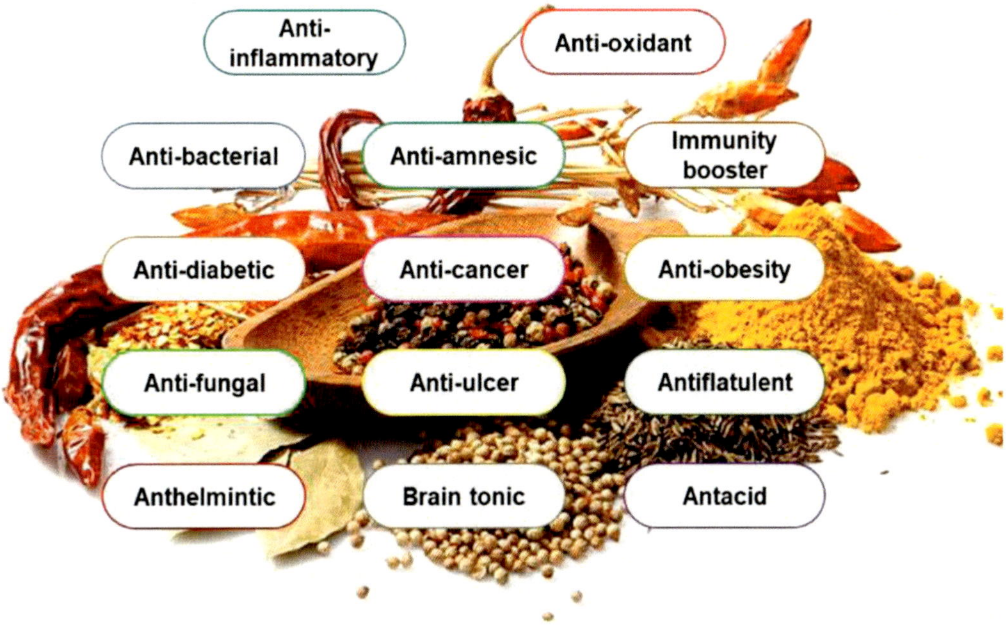

Fig. (1). Different therapeutic activities of Indian spices.

The impact of curcumin on the insulin receptor and beta cell activity brings about changes in human insulin therapy, suggesting careful consideration of incorporating Indian spice therapy into diabetes treatment and insulin delivery. The connection between diabetes, mitochondrial dysfunction, and Indian spices underscores the need to thoroughly evaluate insulin therapy, combining it with hyperglycaemic mitochondrial apoptosis treatment. Turmeric, a spice commonly used in Indian traditional medicine and as a cosmetic, has been employed for wound healing, rheumatoid arthritis, gastrointestinal issues, deworming, and rhinitis. Recent studies in India have focused on its potential to prevent pre-carcinogenic effects, as well as its anti-inflammatory and anti-atherosclerotic properties in biological systems, both in animals and humans. In rats, both turmeric and curcumin have been found to enhance detoxifying enzymes, prevent DNA damage, improve DNA repair, reduce mutations and tumor formation, and exhibit antioxidative capabilities. These therapeutic and preventive benefits of turmeric have been associated with various molecular targets. Additionally, fenugreek seeds, a high-fiber meal commonly used in Indian cuisine, have been shown to lower blood glucose and lipids, making them a potential dietary adjuvant for diabetes management. Similarly, garlic, onions, and ginger have been discovered to positively influence the process of carcinogenesis. Indian spices have been staples in kitchens since ancient times, meeting daily nutritional needs, and have also been employed in traditional medicine. This chapter explores the applications of various Indian spices, as well as their nutritional and physiological benefits. Importantly, these spices have demonstrated positive effects on bodily functions that extend beyond basic nutritional requirements.

1.1. Biological Activities of Spices

Numerous plants possess medicinal advantages and are commonly utilized as spices. The taste of Indian cuisine primarily relies on these spices, which impart flavors like sweetness, spiciness, sourness, and bitterness. Beyond their culinary role, all spices also offer therapeutic properties, promoting wellness and aiding in treating ailments, according to Ayurveda, the Indian school of medicine. Typically, these spices are consumed orally in the form of powders or decoctions. The effectiveness of each spice's therapeutic properties depends on the potency of the specific plant parts that interact with different bodily systems, such as digestion and respiration. Therefore, Ayurveda recommends using particular plant components for specific diseases. Various factors, such as soil conditions, rainfall, altitude, cultivation methods, harvesting, storage, and transportation, significantly impact herbal remedies' true potency and medicinal value. Traditional medicinal benefits are derived from the active chemical constituents found in specific plant parts, and scientific research has explored the pharmacological properties of major Indian spices.

The main objective of this chapter was to underscore the traditional therapeutic uses of common Indian spices, with particular attention to their antimicrobial and antiviral properties. Fig. (**2**) presents several prevalent applications of these spices. Generally, these herbs and spices contain compounds such as polyphenols, flavanols/flavonoids, quinines, alkaloids, polypeptides, or their oxygen-substituted derivatives. Turmeric, for instance, comprises approximately 235 compounds, mainly phenolics and terpenoids, including twenty-two diarylheptanoids, diaryl pentanoids, eight phenylpropenes, and other phenolics [8]. Among these compounds, Curcuminoids like curcumin and monoterpenes play vital roles in various biological activities such as neuroprotection, anti-cancer, antimicrobial, anti-inflammatory, and cardioprotective effects [9]. Clove has been identified as the richest source of flavonoids compared to caraway, coriander, and rosemary [10]. The most biologically active compound in clove is eugenol, which exhibits antibacterial, antiviral, fungicidal, anti-tumor, and dental analgesic properties [11]. Some articles suggest that cardamom and coriander also serve as good sources of flavonoids and act as scavengers of free radicals [12].

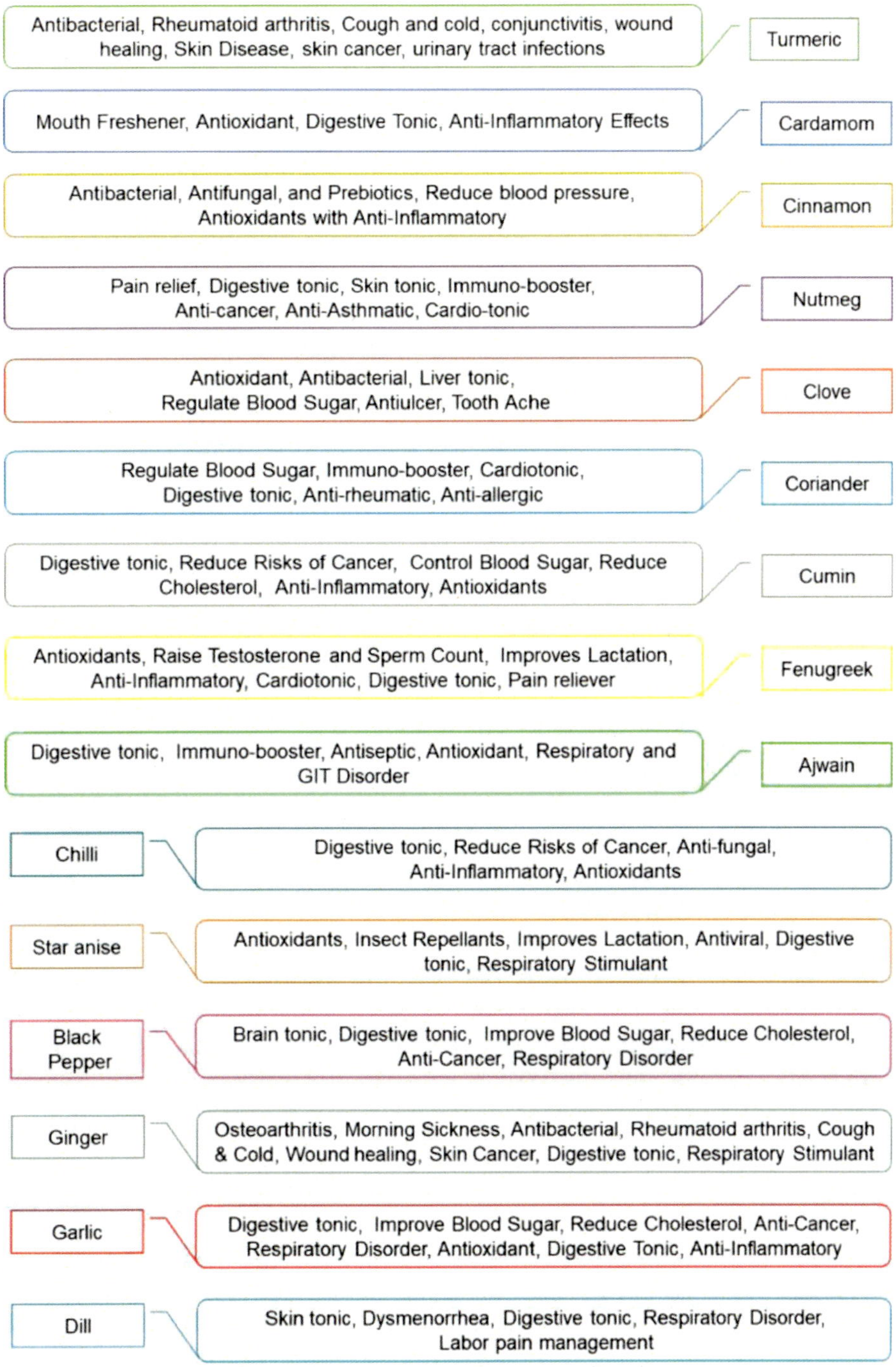

Fig. (2). Multi-therapeutic action of Indian spices.

The roles of black pepper and cardamom aqueous extracts encompass antimicrobial, anti-inflammatory, hypolipidemic, anti-mutagenic, and anti-carcinogenic properties [13, 14]. These extracts contain piperine and eugenol, respectively, which have been found to enhance proliferative signaling pathways in splenocytes, resulting in a potent immunomodulatory effect [15].

Ginger, an oleoresin, contains gingerol and shogaols as its main constituents, which offer a wide array of health benefits. These include antioxidant, anti-inflammatory, antimicrobial, anticancer, neuroprotective, cardiovascular protective, respiratory protective, antiobesity, antidiabetic, antinausea, and antiemetic activities [16]. Notably, inhaling ginger essence has been shown to reduce nausea intensity and emesis episodes following nephrectomy in patients [17]. In animal studies, dill essential oil, when orally administered to rats daily at different doses for two weeks, demonstrated a dose-dependent reduction in total cholesterol, triglyceride, and low-density lipoprotein cholesterol (LDL-C), while increasing high-density lipoprotein cholesterol (HDL-C) [18]. Additionally, the hydroalcoholic dill seed extract showed significant anti-inflammatory and pain-relieving effects in rats [19]. Dill oil and diclofenac-gel exhibited a notable reduction in paw volume in rats when compared to the control group. Remarkably, Dill oil showed an even more significant decrease in paw volume compared to diclofenac [20]. In a study conducted by Sayyah and colleagues, they examined the impact of aqueous and ethanol extracts of dill on the female reproductive system using 56 Wistar female rats. The findings revealed that treatment with a high dose of dill extract significantly prolonged the estrous cycle, estrus phase, and progesterone concentration. Additionally, they investigated the antinociceptive effects of Laurus nobilis essential oil in C-Reflex and spinal Wind-Up models in rats, suggesting that the essential oil, particularly at higher doses (0.06 mg/kg), produced a clear antinociceptive effect, completely abolishing the spinal wind-up while leaving the C-reflex unaffected [21]. Moreover, the anticonvulsant properties of laurel leaf essential oil were evaluated against experimentally induced seizures in mice using maximal electroshock or pentylenetetrazole. The study revealed that certain essential oil components, such as methyl eugenol, eugenol, and pinene, offered protection against seizures [21]. Various studies conducted on animals and humans across the globe have highlighted the numerous health benefits of Cinnamon. These benefits include anti-inflammatory properties, antimicrobial activity, reduced risk of cardiovascular disease, improved cognitive function, and a lowered likelihood of colonic cancer [22]. Historically, Garlic has been used by herbalists during the plague. Louis Pasteur (1822-1895 CE) later discovered its bacteria-killing properties, and it was even applied on battlefields to prevent gangrene [23]. Ajwain extract, known for its antiseptic effect, has been used externally to treat skin infections and has shown promise in this regard [24, 25]. Additionally,

Ajwain extracts are employed for respiratory and digestive infections. Mustard and garlic, containing volatile sulfur compounds, have demonstrated activity against bacterial, fungal, and viral infections [26]. Furthermore, research has indicated that fruit and seed cardamom extracts are rich in volatile compounds that exhibit potent activity against periodontal infection. These extracts have also shown the ability to significantly decrease the secretion of IL-1b, TNF-a, and IL-8 by lipopolysaccharide-stimulated macrophages, thus demonstrating anti-inflammatory activity. Fig. (**3**) provides an overview of some of the important mechanisms through which these spices exert their therapeutic actions.

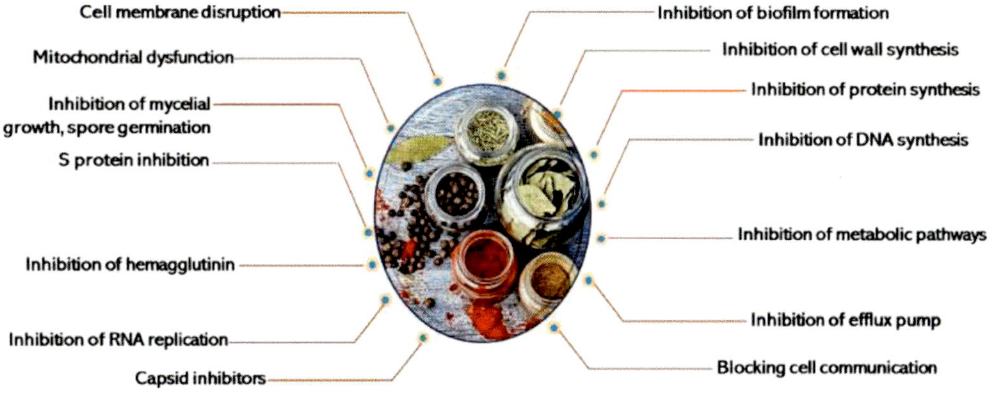

Fig. (3). Mechanism of action of Indian spices.

1.2. Overview of Selected Spices

In this chapter, we try to cover the anti-microbial properties of routinely used spices and herbs in the Indian kitchen. Selected spices mainly belong to the volatile oil class from Fennel, Coriander, Dill, Ajwain, and Cumin, known as umbelliferous fruits. Ginger and turmeric belong to the oleoresin category, while Chili comes from resin. Cardamom, Clove, Cinnamon, Sweet neem, Star anise, Black pepper, Mint leaves, Bay leaves, Basil leaves, Garlic, and Nutmeg also possess a good amount of volatile oils.

Fenugreek contains terpenoids, while mustard and garlic contain sulfur compounds known as sinigrin and allicin, respectively. Eugenol, which possesses potent antimicrobial properties and is effective against periodontal infections, is predominantly found in clove, basil leaves, mint leaves, bay leaves, black pepper, and cinnamon bark. Volatile oil-containing spices also serve as insect repellents. Among all the spices mentioned, the most volatile oil exhibits antibacterial, antifungal, and antiviral properties. *Staphylococcus aureus* (*S. aureus*) and *Candida albicans* (*C. albicans*), common pathogens responsible for the blood-stream and hospital-acquired infections, can be effectively targeted by these

Indian spices. During the ongoing COVID-19 pandemic, many people turn to Kadha, an herbal concoction containing several of these kitchen spices, for its potential benefits.

1.3. Indian Kitchen Spices

1.3.1. Clove Bud

Clove, derived from the flower bud of *Eugenia caryophyllus* or *Syzygium aromaticum* belonging to the *Myrtaceae* family (Fig. **4**), is primarily produced in Zanzibar, Pemba (now part of Tanzania), and Indonesia. In India, clove cultivation is predominant in the hilly regions of Tamil Nadu, Kerala, and Karnataka. The main components of clove are found in its volatile oil, including eugenol (83.13%), β caryophyllene (6.88%), α humulene (2.48%), oxicaryophylene (3.59%), and eugenyl acetate (2.41%) [27]. Clove essential oil serves as an oral antiseptic in combating infections [27]. It demonstrates antimicrobial properties against various strains, such as *S. aureus, E. coli, P. aeruginosa, S. pyogenes, Corynebacterium, S. bacteroides, and C. albicans*, at different concentrations [28]. Additionally, eugenol, a key component of clove, exhibits antiviral effects against herpes viruses HSV-1 and HSV-2 [29].

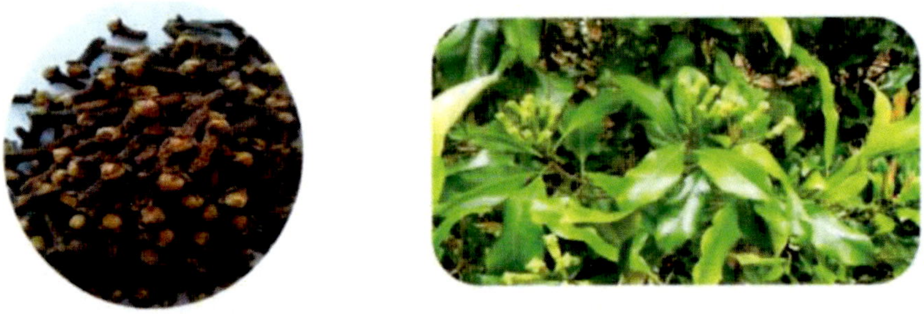

Clove **Clove plant**

Fig. (4). Clove flower bud and plant.

Mechanism: Both eugenol and clove essential oil phenolic compounds are widely recognized for their ability to alter proteins and interact with cell membrane phospholipids, resulting in changes to membrane permeability and inhibition of various types of bacteria and yeast, including gram-negative and gram-positive strains [25].

Eugenol's anti-bacterial properties stem from multiple mechanisms, such as preventing biofilm formation and suppressing the expression of virulence factors in *S. aureus* [30] and *E. coli* [31]. A study reported that the aqueous extract of

Syzygium aromaticum seeds displayed antibacterial effects against *E. coli, P. aeruginosa, and S. aureus*, primarily through effects on membrane permeability and oxidative stress [32].

1.3.2. Cinnamon Bark

Cinnamon serves primarily as a spice, flavoring agent, and food seasoning in India. It belongs to the *Lauraceae* family (Fig. **5**). Among the 250 species of cinnamon, only four are commercially utilized: Ceylon cinnamon (*Cinnamomum verum or Cinnamomum zeylanicum*) from India and Sri Lanka's Ceylon region, Chinese cinnamon (*Cinnamomum cassia or Cinnamomum aromaticum*), Indonesian cinnamon (*Cinnamomum burmannii*), and Vietnamese cinnamon (*Cinnamomum loureiroi*) [33]. Cinnamon bark is abundant in volatile oils and other derivatives, including cinnamic acid, cinnamic aldehyde, cinnamyl acetate, α-cubebene, terpineol, α-cubebene, eugenol, and coumarin [34]. Studies have demonstrated that the essential oils from Cinnamomum cassia bark possess significant inhibitory effects against multi-drug resistant pathogens such as *E. coli, P. aeruginosa, and S. aureus* [35, 36]. Similarly, *Cinnamomum zeylanicum* volatile oil has shown antiviral activity against H1N1 and HSV1 [37, 38]. The main chemical constituents of *C. zeylanicum* are cinnamic aldehyde and eugenol, which exhibit fungicidal activity against *Candida albicans* and other Candida species [39]. Moreover, cinnamaldehyde, a major component in cinnamon, has been found to significantly inhibit neutrophils, macrophages, and total cell numbers in the bronchoalveolar lavage fluid. Treatment with cinnamaldehyde has also led to decreased levels of inflammatory cytokines such as TNF-α, IL-6, IL-13, and IL-1β [40].

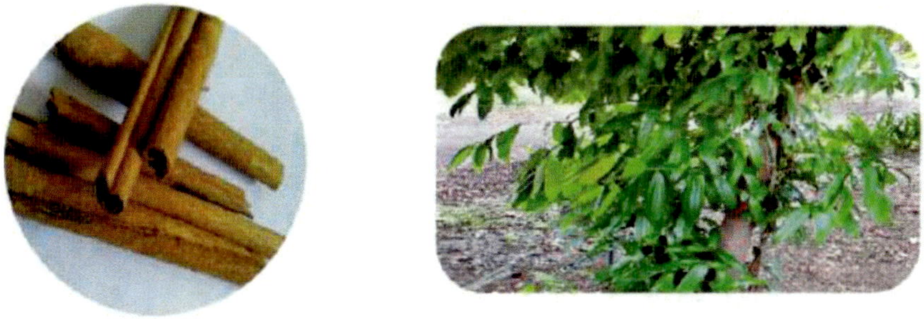

Cinnamon **Cinnamon plant**

Fig. (5). Cinnamon bark and plant.

Mechanism: As per a certain hypothesis, cinnamon bark oil can harm bacterial membranes by disrupting the potassium cation (K^+) gradient. This disturbance leads to a breakdown of the permeability barrier, resulting in the mortality of the cells [41]. Another study focusing on its antifungal properties found that cinnamon oil can enter cell walls and membranes to inflict damage. This, in turn, affects the production of mannan and chitin-glucan [42]. Moreover, the damage caused to cell walls can result in mechanical harm. Consequently, cell metabolism and the activity of specific enzymes are impacted, leading to interference with the synthesis of nucleic acids and proteins. This sequence of events eventually causes further damage to cell nuclei, leading to cell rupture and, ultimately cell death [43].

1.3.3. Cardamom

Cardamom, scientifically known as *Elletaria cardamomum* and belonging to the *Zingiberaceae* family (Fig. **6**), is derived from dried ripe fruit and originates from the evergreen rain forests in the Western Ghats of South India. It is commonly cultivated in the Indian states of Kerala, Karnataka, and Tamil Nadu. An analysis of cardamom oil using GC-MS revealed the presence of significant bioactive chemicals, including terpinyl acetate (38.4%), 1,8-cineole (28.71%), linalool acetate (8.42%), sabinene (5.21%), and linalool (3.97%), which contribute to its various medicinal properties and applications [46]. In India, cardamom serves multiple purposes, acting as a folk medicine, spice, food preservative, and flavor enhancer. Traditionally, it has been utilized as an aromatic stimulant, carminative, astringent, diuretic, anti-inflammatory agent, and treatment for asthma, cardiac disorders, indigestion, rectal diseases, and congestive jaundice. Additionally, cardamom is used as an insect-controlling agent [44, 45]. Notably, a study demonstrated that cardamom's essential oil exhibited effectiveness against *Staphylococcus aureus*, *Salmonella typhi*, *Escherichia coli*, *Streptococci mutans*, and *Candida albicans* fungi [46]. This supports its historical use for the prevention and control of various infections.

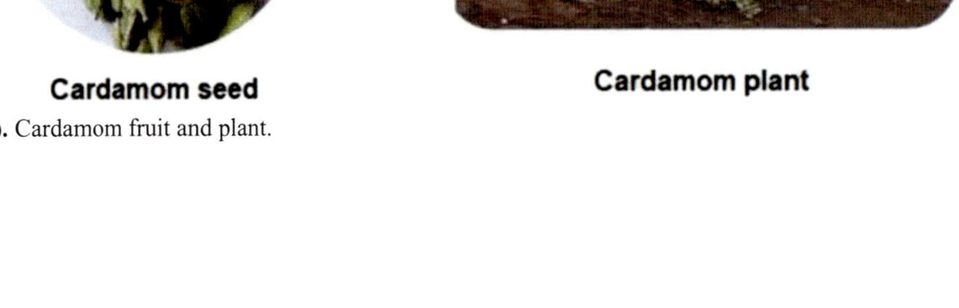

Cardamom seed **Cardamom plant**

Fig. (6). Cardamom fruit and plant.

Mechanism: Cardamom oil possesses an antimicrobial effect due to its main chemical constituent, 1, 8-cineole, which causes cell shrinkage and damages the cell membrane, leading to cell death [47]. Cardamom is rich in phenolic and flavonoid components that may exhibit biological activity [48]. Through HPLC analysis, it has been found that the ethanol extract of cardamom contains (−)-epicatechin, vanillin, p-coumaric acid, trans-ferulic acid, and ellagic acid, all of which demonstrate strong anti-inflammatory and antioxidant properties. Research from the literature reveals that the major constituents of cardamom include α-terpinyl acetate, α-terpineol, 1,8-cineole, and limonene, which potentially affect metabolic syndrome. These terpenes have been shown to reduce blood pressure in normotensive rats and induce endothelium-dependent vasorelaxation in male Wistar rats [49].

1.3.4. Black Pepper

The Genus Piper comprises over 1000 species, including Black pepper, renowned as the 'king of spices' due to its pungent component called piperine. Its botanical name is *Piper nigrum L.* (Fig. **7**), and it belongs to the *Piperaceae* family [50]. Originating from the Western Ghats of India, this distinctive flavor is native to the region. The primary regions for cultivating black pepper in India are Kerala, Tamil Nadu, Karnataka, Konkan, Pondicherry, and the Nicobar Islands [51, 52]. Research has shown that fresh pepper contains phenolic compounds and volatile oil, which can inhibit the growth of various microorganisms, such as *Salmonella typhimurium, Escherichia coli, Staphylococcus aureus, Bacillus subtilis, Pseudomonas aeruginosa, Alternaria alternata, Aspergillus niger, Aspergillus flavus,* and *Fusarium oxysporum.*

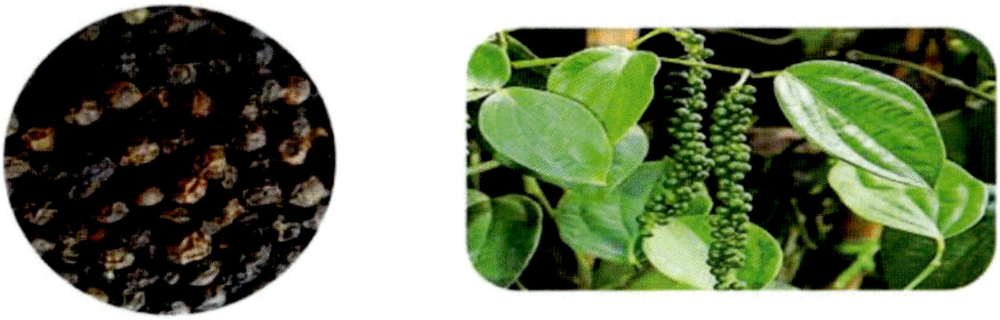

Black pepper seed **Black pepper plant**

Fig. (7). Black pepper and plant.

When tested on HeLa cell lines, Piperine, a primary chemical compound found in black pepper, demonstrated antiviral effects against vesicular stomatitis, Indiana virus, and Human para influenza viruses [53]. Through *in silico* molecular docking studies, it was discovered that piperine exhibited significant inhibitory activity against SARS-COV-2 [54], as well as Ebola and dengue viruses [55], making it a potent inhibitor for these viruses.

Mechanism: The active elements in black pepper hindered cellular respiration by interrupting the tricarboxylic acid (TCA) pathway. This disruption caused the buildup of pyruvic acid and decreased ATP levels, indicating that the chloroform extract of black pepper can alter cell membrane permeability, disrupt bacterial respiratory metabolism, and ultimately result in cell shrinkage and death [56]. Furthermore, the researcher proved that the replication of viruses could be obstructed by targeting the receptor-binding domain (RBD) of the SARS-CoV-2 spike protein and the main protease of SARS-CoV-2 [54].

1.3.5. Coriander

In the Indian culinary realm, Coriander leaves serve as a delightful embellishment for various food dishes, while its seeds are primarily employed as spices and flavor enhancers. Botanically known as *Coriandrum sativum*, this herb belongs to the *Umbelliferae* family (Fig. **8**). India takes the lead in producing around 80% of the world's total coriander seed yield. The major cultivation regions in India include Rajasthan, Madhya Pradesh, Uttar Pradesh, and Southern States like Andhra Pradesh, Karnataka, and Tamil Nadu [57]. Coriander boasts a composition primarily consisting of linalool (57–72%), limonene (0.3–3.7%), α-pinene (1.63–4.81%), β-pinene (0.1– 0.6%), camphene (0.1–0.92%), myrcene (0.18–1.3%), sabinene (0.1–0.3%), camphor (0.2–6.4%), geranyl acetate (1.0–5.0%), and linalyl acetate (1.25–7.1%), alongside other terpene hydrocarbons and terpenoids [58 - 60]. Notably, coriander oil exhibits antimicrobial properties, combating both gram-positive and gram-negative bacteria, dermatophytes, filamentous fungi, and certain yeasts [61]. Additionally, coriander has shown efficacy against Human Immunodeficiency Virus-1 and HIV-2 (HIV-1 and HIV-2).

Mechanism: Coriander oil possesses bactericidal properties by causing the permeabilization of the bacterial membrane. This leads to a complete loss of cellular functions, including metabolic activity, membrane polarization, and efflux activity, all occurring within just 30 minutes of exposure [62]. Moreover, the oil displays antifungal effects against *C. albicans* even at concentrations below the minimum inhibitory level by inhibiting germ tube formation. Additionally, the oil targets the fungal membrane, initiating membrane permeabilization after a 30-minute contact period, resulting in the leakage of significant cellular components such as DNA [63].

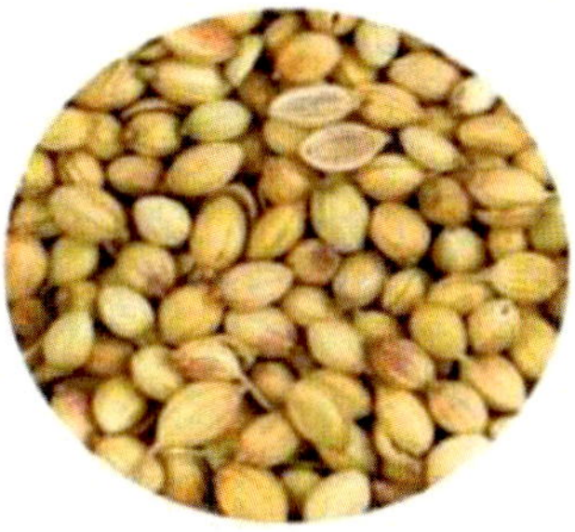

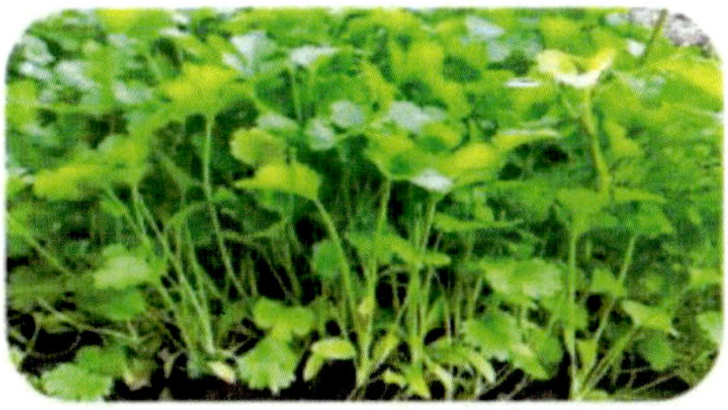

Coriander seed **Coriander plant**

Fig. (8). Coriander fruit and plant.

1.3.6. Fennel

Foeniculum vulgare , commonly known as fennel (Fig. **9**) and belonging to the family *Apiaceae / Umbelliferae*, is widely used in India as a spice, flavoring agent, and a key component of mukhwas (Mouth freshener). Originally native to Southern Europe and the Mediterranean region, it has become one of the popular seed spices in India, mainly cultivated during the Rabi season. Over time, it spread to the Far East and far north of Europe. The major fennel-producing states in India include Gujarat, Rajasthan, Karnataka, Maharashtra, U.P., Punjab, and Bihar. Fennel is highly valued for its nutritional content, being a rich source of vitamins A, B, C, and K, as well as calcium, iron, zinc, sodium, essential and nonessential amino acids, fatty acids, and various polyphenolics, such as neochlorogenic acid, chlorogenic acid, gallic acid, caffeic acid, p-coumaric acid, ferulic acid-7-o-glucoside, quercetin-7-o-glucoside, ferulic acid, 1,5 dicaffeoylquinic acid, hesperidin, cinnamic acid, rosmarinic acid, quercetin, and apigenin [64, 65]. Furthermore, the volatile oil of fennel fruit contains several compounds, including P-anisaldehyde, trans-anethole, (+)-fenchone, (-)-fenchone, thymol, and estragol. Fennel has been evaluated for its potential anti-inflammatory, antimicrobial, antiviral, and antistress properties [66]. Notably, studies have shown that the essential oil of *F. vulgare* exhibits activity against various bacterial strains, such as *Bacillus cereus, Bacillus megaterium, Bacillus subtilis, Bacillus pumilus, Escherichia coli, Klebsiella pneumonia, Micrococcus luteus, Pseudomonas putida, Pseudomonas syringae,* and *Candida albicans* [67]. Moreover, it has demonstrated strong antiviral effects against the DNA virus Herpes simplex type-1 (HSV-1) and the RNA virus parainfluenza type-3 (PI-3) [68]. Additionally, fennel exhibits potent antifungal action against various fungal species, including *Aspergillus niger, Fusarium oxysporum, Alternaria alternata, Candida albicans, Rhizoctonia solani, Mucor rouxii, and Aspergillus flavus* [69 - 71].

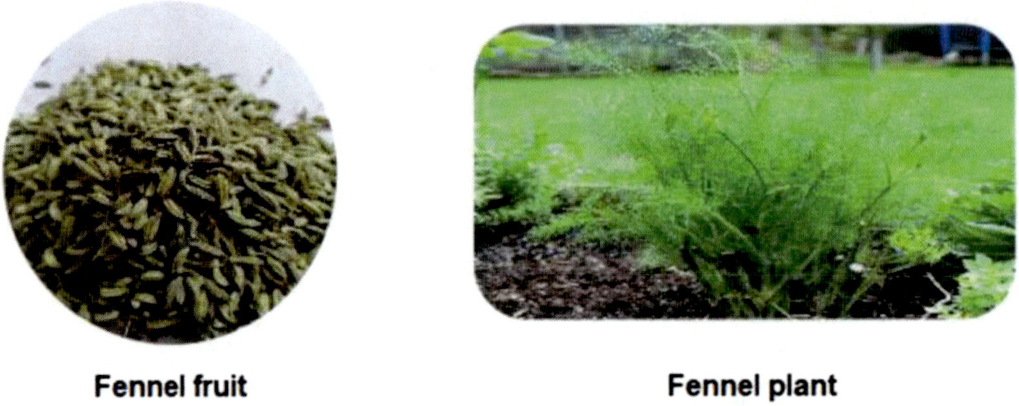

Fig. (9). Fennel fruit and plant.

Mechanism: The essential oil significantly impacts the integrity of cell membranes, causing the release of electrolytes and the subsequent loss of cellular contents, which ultimately results in bactericidal effects [72]. Fennel essential oil exhibits antifungal properties, causing harm to both the plasma membrane and internal cell structures, potentially inhibiting key mitochondrial enzymes, including succinate dehydrogenase, malate dehydrogenase, and ATPase [73]. The primary chemical constituent, trans-anethole, plays a crucial role in inhibiting the later stages of the HSV-1 lifecycle by specifically targeting the redox signaling pathway [74].

1.3.7. Cumin

Cumin, derived from the fruit of *Cuminum cyminum* in the *Apiaceae* family (Fig. **10**), is a volatile oil extensively used as a spice and flavor enhancer in Indian cuisine. It has become a fundamental ingredient in Indian curries and is utilized in various dishes such as Jeera Paratha, Jeera Rice, and Masala Buttermilk [75]. Originally hailing from the Mediterranean and northern Africa, cumin is now predominantly cultivated in India. A study comparing microwave and conventionally roasted cumin oils showed similar antimicrobial properties against *E. coli, S. aureus, P. aeruginosa, A. niger, A. parasiticus*, and *C. albicans* using the disk diffusion method. Notably, the roasted oils exhibited stronger antimicrobial effects than the raw oils [76]. Furthermore, Sheikh investigated the antibacterial effects of cumin extracts on several gram-positive and gram-negative bacteria. The research revealed that cumin seed extracts, with very low minimum inhibitory concentrations (MIC), could potentially control *Escherichia coli, Bacillus subtilis, Klebsiella pneumonia,* and *Staphylococcus aureus* [77]. The primary components found in all cumin oils were monoterpenes such as -pinene, p-cymene, and -terpinene, along with terpenoid aldehydes like cuminic aldehyde and the isomeric menthadien carboxaldehyde [75]. Additionally, cumin is a rich source of iron, a vital mineral for supporting immune health. A specific isolated component called 1-(2-Ethyl, 6-Heptyl) Phenol found in cumin demonstrated significant antiviral effects against HAV, Cox B4, and HSV1, as well as antidermatophytic effects against *Microsporum* and *Epidermophyton* and *Trichophyton spp.* at remarkably low concentrations of 6.25 and 12.5 μg/mL [78].

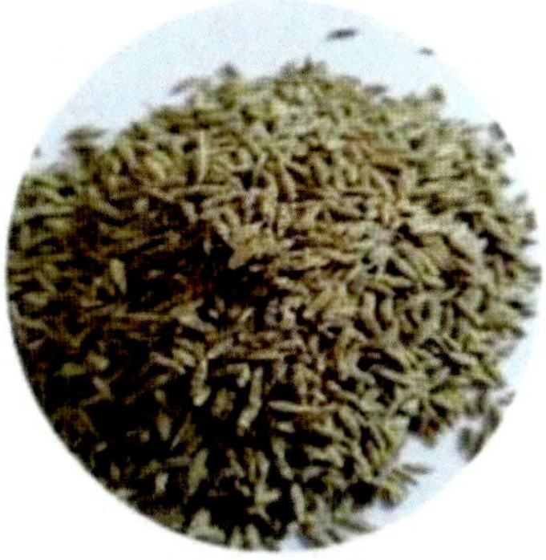

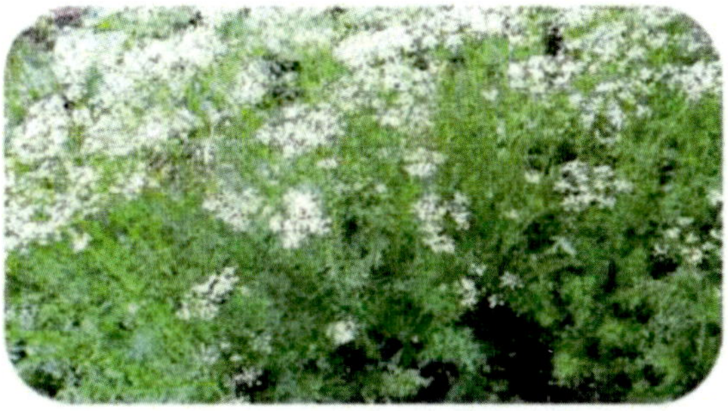

Cummin seed **Cummin plant**

Fig. (10). Cumin seed and plant.

Mechanism: Much research has suggested that the antiviral effect could be attributed to phenol. This compound interacts with the vero cell membrane and/or the HSV-1 envelope [78, 79]. Another study utilized TLC-bioautography to show that cuminaldehyde, a prominent bioactive constituent found in *C. cyminum*, displays potent antibacterial properties against various bacteria such as *Bacillus cereus, Staphylococcus aureus, Escherichia coli,* and *Salmonella typhi* [80].

1.3.8. Dill

The herb dill, scientifically known as *Anethum graveolens L.* and belonging to the *Apiaceae* family (Fig. **11**), yields leaves and seeds. Another variety of dill called Anethum Sowa is found in India. Sowa is primarily grown as a cold crop in India, its subcontinent, Japan, and the Malaysian archipelago [81]. The fresh and preserved leaves serve as condiments and make tea, while the seeds are used as a spice. Aromatic plants like dill play a vital role in enhancing the flavor of various dishes, including pickles, sauces, salads, and soups [82, 83]. In Gujarat, India, fresh dill leaves are commonly used to make a dish called 'Sabji.' Medicinally, dill seeds are a key ingredient in gripe water given to infants to relieve colic pain and flatulence in young children [84]. Long-term preserved dill seed oil contains a significant amount of D-carvone (50.1 percent) and D-limonene (44.1 percent), with carvone (71.0 percent) being the primary compound. Dill seeds also contain trace amounts of carveol, dihydrocarvones, and R-phellandrene, which are primarily found in dill leaf oils [85]. In a study on the antimicrobial activity of dill seed essential oil against four gram-positive bacteria (*S. aureus, Bacillus cereus, Enterococcus faecalis,* and *L. monocytogenes*), and four gram-negative bacteria (*E. coli, Yersinia enterocolitica*), dill essential oil demonstrated good to average activity. The largest inhibition zones (15 mm) and MICs (0.62 mg/mL) were observed against *S. aureus and V. cholerae* [86, 87]. Moreover, dill oil exhibited anti-mycotic and anti-mycotoxigenic properties, inhibiting the growth of different fungi, including *Aspergillus flavus, Aspergillus parasiticus, Aspergillus ochraceus, Penicillium verrucosum, Fusarium graminearum,* and *Aspergillus niger*, at a concentration of 5 mg/mL [88].

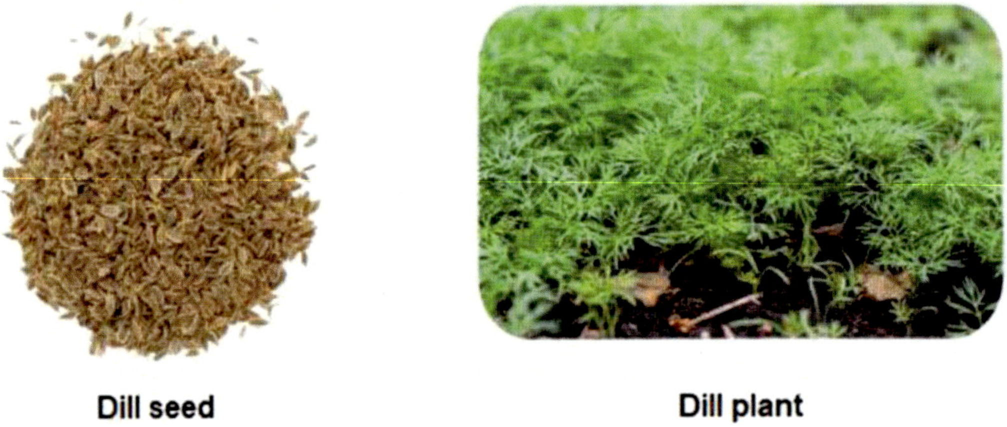

Fig. (11). Dill fruit and plant.

Mechanism: According to research, dill essential oils have been proposed to interact with the lipid components of cell membranes. This interaction can have two possible outcomes: either they increase ion permeability, leading to the leakage of cell components, or they can harm bacterial enzymes responsible for polysaccharide synthesis [89]. The presence of monoterpenes in the essential oil plays a crucial role in damaging the bacterial cell membrane due to their lipophilic nature [90]. There are several hypotheses regarding dill's anti-fungal effect. Some suggest that certain components in dill may disrupt the enzymatic cell system, affecting fungi's energy generation and synthesis of structural compounds [91, 92]. Another possibility is that the active components could cause the denaturation of enzymes responsible for spore germination or interfere with the amino acids required for spore germination [93]. Lastly, it is also suggested that dill exposure to different volatile substances might cause irreversible damage to the fungal cell membrane, cell wall, and cellular organelles [94, 95].

1.3.9. Ocimum (Tulsi or Holy Basil)

Ocimum sanctum , commonly known as Tulsi or Holy Basil, is a plant belonging to the *Lamiaceae* family (Fig. **12**). Revered for its medicinal properties, it is often referred to as the "Queen of plants" and the "mother medicine of nature" due to its perceived healing attributes [96]. Basil's diverse chemical components have been utilized to address various health conditions, including viral ocular, respiratory, and hepatic infections. Noteworthy medicinal compounds found in basil include monoterpenoids like fenchone, carvone, cineole, geraniol, linalool, and thujone, sesquiterpenoids such as caryophyllene and farnesol, flavonoids like apigenin, and a vital anti-viral element known as ursolic acid (a triterpenoid) [97]. Basil leaves have been shown to combat three periodontal pathogens, namely *Aggregatibacter actinomycetemcomitans, Prevotella intermedia, and Porphyromonas gingivalis* [98]. The essential oil derived from basil demonstrates the potential to be an effective topical antimicrobial agent against skin infections caused by *S. aureus, P. aeruginosa,* and *E. coli* [99]. Additionally, *Ocimum sanctum L.* exhibits anti-microbial properties against various pathogenic microorganisms, including *Staphylococcus aureus, Bacillus pumius, Pseudomonas aeruginosa, Bacillus subtilis,* and *Escherichia coli* [100, 101]. Ursolic acid has been observed to inhibit viral infections caused by herpes simplex virus (HSV)-1 and human immunodeficiency virus (HIV), as well as tumor growth [102]. Numerous studies have demonstrated that basil leaf extracts in aqueous and methanol form, as well as basil seed oil, enhance the immune response by increasing T-helper cells and natural killer cells, lymphocyte count, phagocytic activity, neutrophil count, antibody titer, and more, serving as a defense mechanism against various infections [103 - 105]. Furthermore, research indicates that basil leaf oil possesses antifungal activity against several fungi strains, including *Aspergillus flavus and toxin-producing species of penicillin-like P. aurantiogriseum, P. brevicimpactum, P. chrysogenum, P. glabrum, P. expansum, P. nordicum, P. rugulosum, P. sodium, P. verrucosum*, and others [107]. It has also shown efficacy against Candida species, such as *C. albicans* and *C. tropicalis*, which cause candidiasis [108].

Mechanism: According to a report, tulsi was found to have an immunomodulatory effect by increasing the levels of interferon, interleukin 4, and T helper cells, which can enhance the body's response to infections [109]. A molecular docking study was conducted on three chemical constituents in tulsi: vicenin, sorientin 4'-O-glucoside 2''-O-phydroxy-benzoate, and ursolic acid. The study revealed that these constituents can inhibit the main protease of SARS-CoV-2 [110]. Furthermore, the researcher explored the impact of basil leaf extract on bacteria using scanning electron microscopy. The results indicated that the extract caused cell wall degradation, damage to cytoplasmic membrane proteins, protein binding, leakage of cell contents, coagulation of cytoplasm, and depletion of the proton motive force [111].

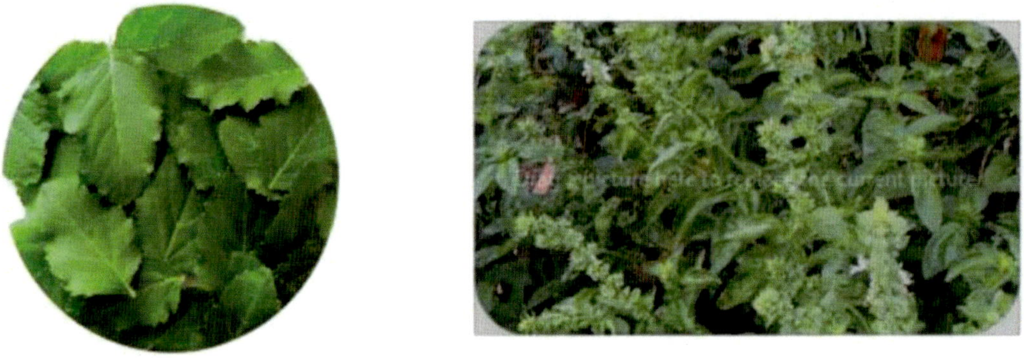

Basil leaves **Basil plant**

Fig. (12). Basil leaves and plant.

1.3.10. Ajwain

Ajwain, a herbaceous plant from the *Apiaceae* family (Fig. **13**), is widely cultivated in Egypt, Iran, Pakistan, Afghanistan, India, and parts of Europe, particularly Gujarat and Rajasthan in India. It is valued for its aromatic and pungent qualities, making it a popular spice used to flavor various food items. The composition of Ajwain includes significant amounts of fiber (11.9%), carbohydrates (38.6%), tannins, glycosides, moisture (8.9%), protein (15.4%), fat (18.1%), saponins, flavone, and mineral matter (7.1%), such as calcium, phosphorous, iron, and nicotinic acid. Notably, Ajwain fruits yield about 2% to 4% of brownish essential oil, primarily composed of thymol (35% to 60%) [112, 113]. Ajwain has been found to possess various beneficial effects, including being antiseptic, stimulant, carminative, diuretic, anesthetic, antimicrobial, antiviral, nematocidal, antiulcer, antihypertensive, antitussive, bronchodilator, antiplatelet, hepatoprotective, and hypolipidemic. It has been subjected to antibacterial testing using acetone and aqueous extracts against several strains, showing higher activity in the acetone extract [114]. Additionally, an ethanolic extract of Ajwain demonstrated antibacterial activity against *Helicobacter pylori* strains [115]. The methanolic extract of Ajwain exhibited bactericidal activity against various bacterial strains, while an alcoholic extract displayed effectiveness against certain fungi [116 - 118]. Furthermore, the antiviral activity of ajwain essential oil was assessed against the Japanese encephalitis virus [119].

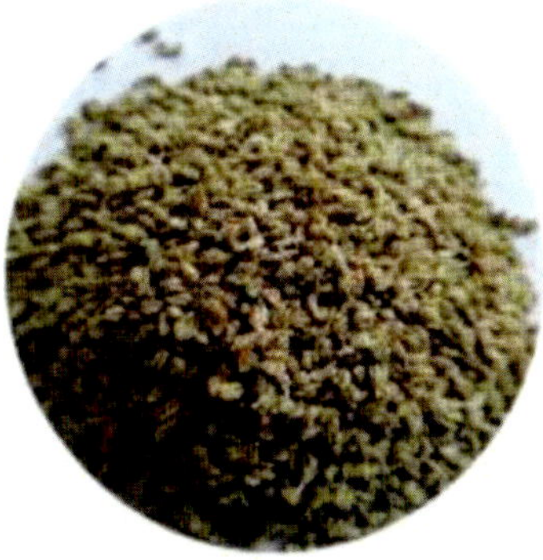

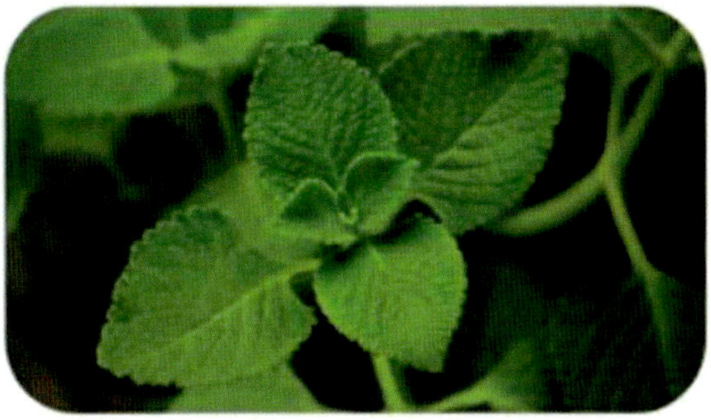

Ajwain seed **Ajwain plant**

Fig. (13). Ajwain fruit and plant.

Mechanism: According to a report, the essential oil of Ajwain may contain significant levels of thymol or carvacrol. These phenolic compounds have been found to exhibit either bactericidal or bacteriostatic properties, depending on their concentration [120]. The study also highlighted that the oil strongly inhibited the growth and spore germination of the toxigenic fungi *A. ochraceus* [121]. Additionally, when a methanolic extract of ajwain was tested using the agar well diffusion method, it showed bactericidal activity against 11 different species at a concentration of 2 mg per well.

The Diameter of Inhibition Zones (DIZ) was measured, and the results showed that the zones of inhibition were larger than 15 mm for *Staphylococcus aureus* and *Staphylococcus epidermidis*, 10–14 mm for *Pseudomonas aeruginosa* and *Bacillus pumilus*, and 7–9 mm for *Escherichia coli, Klebsiella pneumonia*, and *Bordetella bronchiseptica* [116].

1.3.11. Fenugreek

Fenugreek, scientifically known as *Trigonella foenum-graecum Linn. (Fabaceae)*, is a seed spice extensively used to enhance various cuisines' flavor, color, and texture. Additionally, it has been utilized for medicinal purposes in traditional systems [122]. Across different countries, fenugreek leaves and seeds are consumed for a variety of uses, such as medicinal applications like anti-diabetic, blood sugar and cholesterol level reduction, anti-cancer, and antimicrobial effects. It is also used in food preparation, such as flavoring cheese in Switzerland, making stew with rice in Iran, creating syrup and bitter run in Germany, and mixing seed powder with flour for flatbread in Egypt. Fenugreek is also employed as a coffee substitute in Africa, controlling insects in grain storage and perfume industries [123]. The seeds of fenugreek contain b-carotene, while the leaves are a rich source of ascorbic acid. They are also abundant in fiber, calcium, zinc, and iron. Additionally, the seeds contain small amounts of volatile and fixed oil. The plant possesses various ethnomedicinal qualities, including being antimicrobial, laxative, uterine tonic, expectorant, restorative, galactagogue, anti-carcinogenic, anti-inflammatory, anticholesterolemic, antiviral, and antioxidant [123, 124]. Researchers have found that silver nanoparticles derived from fenugreek seeds exhibit antibacterial properties against *Aspergillus flavus*, *Trichophyton rubrum*, and *Trichoderma viridiae*. Ultrasonically produced nanoparticles have shown greater stability, antibacterial activity, and antioxidant properties compared to those produced by magnetic stirring. Fenugreek seed extracts have also demonstrated antibacterial activity against *E. coli* and Staphylococcus bacteria [125]. Various aqueous extracts from different parts of the fenugreek plant, using solvents such as methanol, petroleum ether, and ethyl acetate, have been tested for their action against fungal strains like *Fusarium graminearum, Botrytis cinerea, Alternaria sp., Rhizoctonia solani,* and *Pythium aphanidermatum* [126]. The effectiveness of fenugreek extracts against *Helicobacter pylori*, a bacterium associated with gastric ulcers, has been reported [127]. In the context of COVID-19 treatment, the researcher Dharmashekara analyzed three important proteins encoded by the virus (envelope protein 5 × 29, RNA binding nucleocapsid protein 1SSK, and spike glycoprotein 6ACD) for potential virion accumulation. Trigoneoside IB, a compound derived from Fenugreek, exhibited the highest binding affinity and stable interaction with amino acid residues in the active sites of COVID-19 proteins. Trigoneoside has also been reported to show *in silico* antiviral activity against the Zika virus [129, 130].

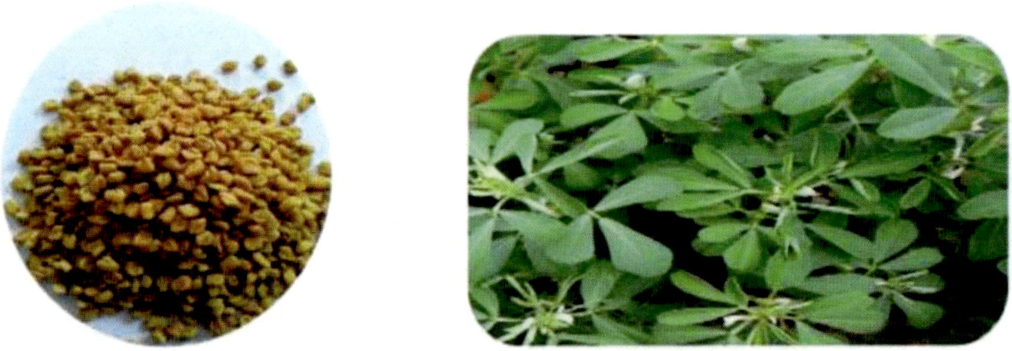

Fenugreek seed **Fenugreek plant**

Fig. (14). Fenugreek seed and plant.

Mechanism: The researcher demonstrated that when combined with silver nanoparticles, the phytochemical constituents have an impact on the cell wall of bacterial pathogens, leading to the release of proteins [131]. It has been reported that pathogenic bacteria release enzymes when experiencing stress or during sporulation. The higher concentration of these enzymes indicates that the silver nanoparticles create an adverse environment for the bacteria, prompting the release of the enzymes.

1.3.12. Mustard

Indian mustard, scientifically known as *Brassica juncea* and belonging to the Brassicaceae family (*Cruciferae*) (Fig. **15**), is primarily cultivated in countries such as Bangladesh, Central Africa, China, India, Japan, Nepal, and Pakistan. It contains several essential components, including fatty oil (30-35%), proteins (40%), phenyl propane derivatives, notably sinapine (choline ester of sinapic acid, 1%), and glucosinolates, primarily sinigrin (allylglucosinolates, 1-5%). Notably, it has exhibited significant antiviral activity against the influenza virus A/H1N1 at a concentration of 1.25 mg/mL of *Brassica juncea* extract, suggesting its potential therapeutic effect against the influenza virus/H1N1 [132]. In another study focused on callus culture derived from mustard hypocotyl explants, a wide range of secondary metabolites were identified, including volatile oil, alkaloids, anthraquinone glycoside, saponin, tannin, and flavonoids [133]. The researchers also investigated the antibacterial properties of the callus extract in both light-induced and dark-induced callus stages of mustard, testing against various microorganisms, such as *E. coli, S. aureus, P. aeruginosa,* and *K. pneumonia.* It was observed that the light-induced callus stages produced higher phenolic content compared to the dark stages and exhibited stronger antibacterial effects.

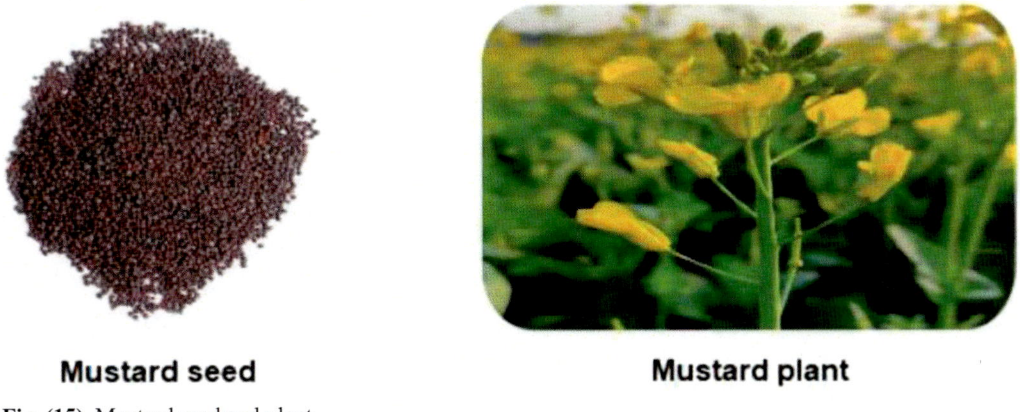

Fig. (15). Mustard seed and plant.

Moreover, a study on *Brassica juncea L.* seed meal and purified polyphenols demonstrated their selective antibacterial effects against *Escherichia coli, Bacillus subtilis, Listeria monocytogenes, Staphylococcus aureus,* and *Pseudomonas fluorescens* [134]. The hydrolyzed extract showed a minimum inhibitory concentration of 0.1 g/L or less. Furthermore, the antimicrobial potential of different extracts (methanol, ethanol, and ethyl acetate) from *Brassica juncea* seeds was evaluated against various bacteria (*Staphylococcus aureus, Bacillus cereus, Escherichia coli, Pseudomonas aeruginosa,* and *Salmonella typhi*) and fungi (*Aspergillus Niger, Mucor mucaralis, Trichophyton tonsurans, Microsporum ferrogenium,* and *Aspergillus flavus* strains) using the agar well diffusion method [135]. This study unveiled the synergistic antimicrobial effect of mustard essential oil and cinnamon essential oil on various bacteria, *Pectobacterium carotovorum*, and *Salmonella enterica* sub sp. enterica, using agar diffusion and vapor diffusion assays. The researchers reported that mustard essential oil exhibited a more potent response compared to cinnamon oil [136].

Mechanism: Some research studies indicated that the use of mustard essential oil led to cell cycle arrest, causing bacterial filamentation. When exposed to concentrations lower than the minimum inhibitory concentration, the bacterial cells exhibited a more elongated and filamentous structure [136]. The extent of this filamentation appeared to be directly related to the concentration of mustard essential oil, as higher levels of the oil resulted in more pronounced filamentous structures at the MIC concentrations.

The reason behind this cell filamentation could be attributed to certain isothiocyanates, such as AITC, which have been observed to induce cell cycle arrest in cells [137]. Furthermore, the isothiocyanate family was shown to impact cell fluidity and homeostatic pressure, leading to visible disruptions in the cell wall [138].

1.3.13. Bay Leaves

Cinnamomum Tamala (Buch-Ham.), a tree belonging to the *Lauraceae* family (Fig. **16**), is indigenous to India, Nepal, Bhutan, and China. It is commonly known as Tejpat, Malabar leaf, and Indian bay leaf in India. The tree reaches a size of up to 1.4 meters in girth and 7.5 meters in height. The parts of the plant utilized are the leaves, bark, and essential oil [139]. The essential oil extracted from the leaves contains furan sesquiterpenoids as its main constituents. Among these, furan ogermenone comprises the highest proportion (59.5%), followed by caryophyllene (6.6%), sabinene (4.8%), germacrene D (4.6%), and curcumenol (2.3%). The leaf oil contains a significant amount of sesquiterpenoids, accounting for 968.8%, with furan sesquiterpenoids making up 79.3% of that total. These furan sesquiterpenoids include furanodienone (46.6%), curzerenone (17.6%), furanodiene (1.8%), and curzerene (1.2%). Notably, the cinnamon leaf oil contains eugenol and cinnamaldehyde, which may cause irritation to local mucous and dermal membranes. Due to its distinctive aroma and peppery flavor, *C. Tamala* has been widely used as a spice in the food industry. The primary constituents of tej patta oil are -linalool (60.73%), -pinene (10.54%), -pinene (10.42%), limonene (3.21%), and camphene (3.16%). There are also trace amounts of eugenol and cinnamaldehyde [140]. Other constituents found in the plant include β-caryophyllene (25.3%), linalool (13.4%), caryophyllene oxide (10.3%), p-cymene, geraniol, benzaldehyde, 1,8-cineole, salicylaldehyde, γ-terpinene, cis-sabinene hydrate, trans-sabinene hydrate, Pinocarvone, borneol, 2-methyl benzofuran, tepinen-4-ol, p-cymen-8-ol, α-terpineol, cinnamaldehyde, carvone, bornyl acetate, cinnamyl alcohol, cinnamyl acetate, β-caryophyllene, cinnamic acid, coumarin, spathulenol, β-copaen-4a-ol, and monoterpenoid hydrocarbons [141]. *Cinnamomum Tamala* possesses various medicinal properties, including hypolipidemic and hypoglycemic effects. It also exhibits potent antibacterial activity against *Escherichia coli, Bacillus subtilis, and Saccharomyces cerevisiae*. In folk medicine, *C. Tamala* has been traditionally used as a brain tonic and anthelmintic, particularly for treating anal and rectal diseases [142]. Additionally, the plant is known for its carminative, diuretic, and anti-flatulent effects and is considered beneficial for heart abnormalities. Both the aqueous and alcoholic extracts of *Cinnamomum Tamala* have demonstrated potential antibacterial activity against several bacterial strains, including *Enterobacter aerogenes, Escherichia coli, Klebsiella pneumonia, Proteus mirabilis, Proteus Vulgaris,* and *Salmonella typhimurium*, belonging to *Enterobacteriaceae*. The alcoholic extract showed higher activity compared to the aqueous extract. *Klebsiella pneumonia* exhibited the highest susceptibility among the tested bacteria, while *Salmonella typhimurium* and *Escherichia coli* were the most resistant [142]. Furthermore, the volatile oil of *C. Tamala* has been found to possess antifungal properties against *Aspergillus Niger, Fusarium moniliforme, A. solani,* and *A. oryzae* [143].

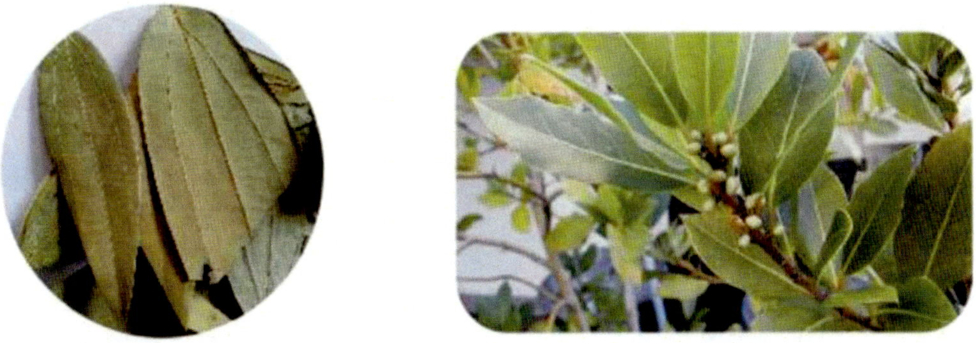

Bay leaves **Bay plant**

Fig. (16). Bay leaves and plant.

Mechanism: Volatile oils and their components possess significant characteristics, such as hydrophobicity. This quality causes an increased partitioning of lipids within bacterial cell membranes and mitochondria, disrupting the cell structure and rendering them more permeable. Consequently, there is a greater leakage of critical molecules and ions from the bacterial cells, ultimately leading to the bacteria's demise [144]. The volatile oil derived from *C. tamala* damages the bacterial cell wall, causing leakage and ultimately resulting in bacterial death [145]. Farisa Banu's research indicates that the essential oil exhibits synergistic effects, effectively inhibiting *Pseudomonas aeruginosa* biofilms [146]. Furthermore, the extract of *C. tamala* leaves displays anti-fungal activity by inhibiting mycelial growth [143].

1.3.14. Chilli

Chilli (*Capsicum annuum L.*), a member of the *Solanaceae* family (Fig. **17**), is the most commonly used and widespread spice in India. India is a leading global producer of chili, with approximately 0.79 million hectares dedicated to its cultivation. Red chilies are popularly used worldwide as a spice due to their pungent taste, vibrant red color, and distinct flavor. Beyond their culinary significance, chilies hold high medicinal value, particularly as an anti-cancer and instant pain relief agent. In various cuisines across the globe, chilies play an integral and crucial role, contributing to pungency, taste, flavor, and color. The pungency in chilies is attributed to the alkaloid Capsaicin present in the placenta connecting the seeds to the pericarp. On the other hand, the red color in chilies is caused by two major carotenoids: capsanthin (35-45%) and capsorubin (6-18%). Chilies are also abundant in proteins, lipids, carbohydrates, fibers, mineral salts (calcium, phosphorus, and iron), and vitamins A, D3, E, C, K, B2, and B12 [147]. The fruits of chili are an excellent source of phytochemical compounds with health benefits. These include ascorbic acid (vitamin C), carotenoids (provitamin A), tocopherols (vitamin E), flavonoids, and capsaicinoids, which play a significant role in preventing chronic diseases such as cancer, asthma, coughs, sore throats, toothache, diabetes, and cardiovascular diseases [148]. Chilies possess antioxidant, anti-mutagenic, hypocholesterolemic, and immunosuppressive properties [147], and they also demonstrate the ability to inhibit bacterial growth and platelet agglomeration. Researchers Soumya and Nair evaluated the antifungal effectiveness of *Capsicum frutescens L.* extracts against seed-borne fungi, including *Aspergillus flavus*, *A. niger*, and *Penicillium sp* [149].

Mechanism: Capsaicinoids and carotenoids are the primary compounds found in peppers, and they hold significant importance and fascination. As alkaloid compounds, capsaicinoids are responsible for the distinctive spiciness of hot chili peppers. These bioactive molecules are exclusively produced in the Capsicum genus and play essential roles in the fields of food, medicine, and even defense weaponry [150]. Prasch's research highlighted that the major components of capsicum, namely capsaicinoids and capsinoids, exhibit favorable antibacterial properties, resistance-modulating effects, and inhibitory actions against *Mycobacterium smegmatis* [151]. Moreover, the methanolic extract of *Capsicum annuum* demonstrated notable antiviral activity against herpes simplex virus types 1 and 2, possibly due to the extract's phytochemical compounds interfering with virus attachment and penetration into cells. It is likely that the primary function of chili is to modify cellular and viral receptors, thus preventing the virus from attaching to cells [152].

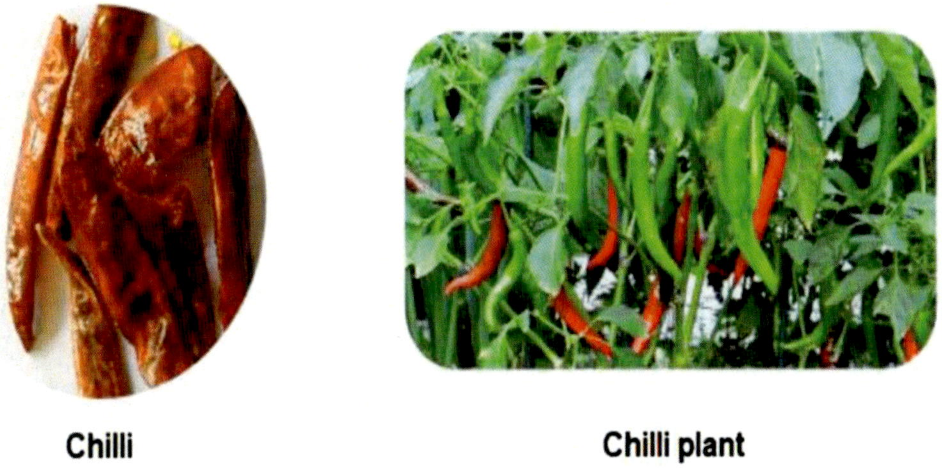

Fig. (17). Chili fruit and plant.

Obi suggests that modifying the receiving cells before the viral infection would significantly decrease the penetration ability of viral cells [153]. Consequently, the viruses would be unable to bind to the receptor, thereby having no impact on the cell. De Lucca's research focused on two saponins, CAY-1 and CAY-2, found in *Capsicum frutescence.* Among them, CAY-1 demonstrated potent anti-fungal properties against 16 distinct fungal strains, including *Aspergillus fumigatus*, by disrupting the membrane integrity of fungal cells [154].

1.3.15. Garlic

Garlic (*Allium sativum L.*) is a fragrant plant belonging to the *Amaryllidaceae* family. It is an annual spice and has been widely used as a medicinal herb since ancient times. This herbaceous plant is consumed worldwide as both a food and a traditional remedy for various ailments. Garlic possesses numerous biological properties, including anticarcinogenic, antioxidant, antidiabetic, renoprotective, anti-atherosclerotic, antibacterial, antifungal, and antihypertensive activities, as recognized in traditional medicine. *A. sativum* contains several sulfur-containing compounds such as alliin, allicin, ajoenes, vinyldithiins, and flavonoids like quercetin. It is considered the second most commonly used Allium species after onions (*Allium cepa* L.), which are employed as a remedy for ailments such as colds, influenza, snake bites, and hypertension. Garlic has also been investigated for its immunomodulatory, anti-inflammatory, and antioxidant properties. Specific constituents found in garlic, such as allyl propyl disulfide, allicin, cysteine sulfoxide, and S-allyl cysteine sulfoxide, have been shown to decrease blood glucose levels. They achieve this by preventing insulin activation caused by the liver, enhancing insulin secretion from pancreatic beta cells, isolating insulin from bonded forms, and increasing cell sensitivity to insulin. *In vitro* studies have demonstrated that aqueous, ethanolic, and dichloromethane extracts of *A. sativum* have anthelmintic activity against *Haemonchus contortus*, with the most effective ethanolic extract. Additionally, the aqueous garlic extract has potent activity against *Trichuris muris* and *Angiostrongylus cantonensis*. Garlic extracts have exhibited antibacterial activity against both Gram-negative (*Kl. pneumonia and E. coli*) and Gram-positive (*e.g.*, *Bacillus subtilis* and *S. aureus*) strains. Methanolic garlic extract has shown antimicrobial activity against all tested strains except *S. aureus* [155]. Researchers have isolated a novel antifungal protein called allivin from *A. sativum*, which demonstrates antifungal activity against *Botrytis cinerea*, *Mycosphaerella arachidicola*, and *Physalosporapiricola* [156]. In an *in vivo* study, antibody-alliinase conjugates and alliin were found to be effective against murine pulmonary aspergillosis [157]. Allicin, a compound present in garlic, has shown antifungal activity against *Candida albicans* [158], *Saccharomyces cerevisiae*, and *Aspergillus fumigatus* in both *in vitro* and *in vivo* experiments [159, 160]. Studies have also shown that garlic extract is effective against viruses such as Newcastle Disease Virus (NDV), HSV-1 and 2, PIV-3, VV, VSV, and HRV-2, among others [161].

Mechanism: Allicin functions by hindering the synthesis of RNA, DNA, and proteins in the parasite. Additionally, garlic-derived phytochemicals like allicin and diallyl trisulfide (DATS) have exhibited antiparasitic effects against various parasites, including *Entamoeba histolytica, Plasmodium falciparum, Babesia, Theleria, Trypanosoma brucei,* and *Giardia lamblia.* Research has shown that aqueous garlic extracts effectively impede lipid synthesis, contributing to their anticandidal properties [162]. *In vitro*, experiments have demonstrated that ajoene, at concentrations below 20 µg/mL, effectively inhibited the growth of both *A. niger* and *C. albicans* [163]. Numerous studies have highlighted the potent antiviral properties of garlic and its organosulfur compounds against various human, animal, and plant pathogenic viruses. Pre-clinical data supports the idea that garlic and its organosulfur compounds exert powerful anti-viral effects through multiple mechanisms, including the blockade of viral entry into host cells, inhibition of reverse transcriptase, RNA polymerase, and DNA synthesis, suppression of immediate early gene 1 transcription, and interference with signaling pathways [164].

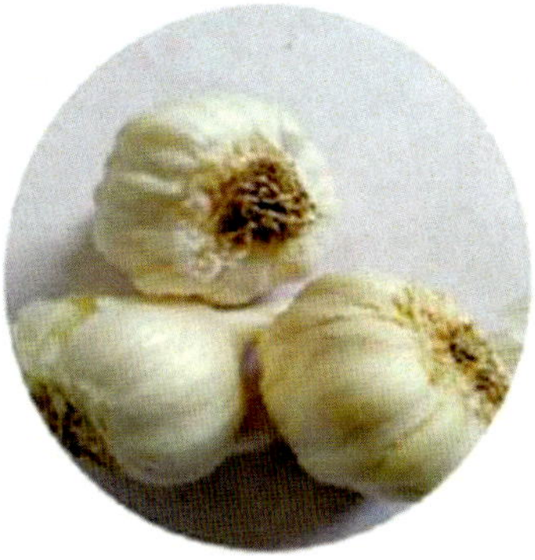

Garlic

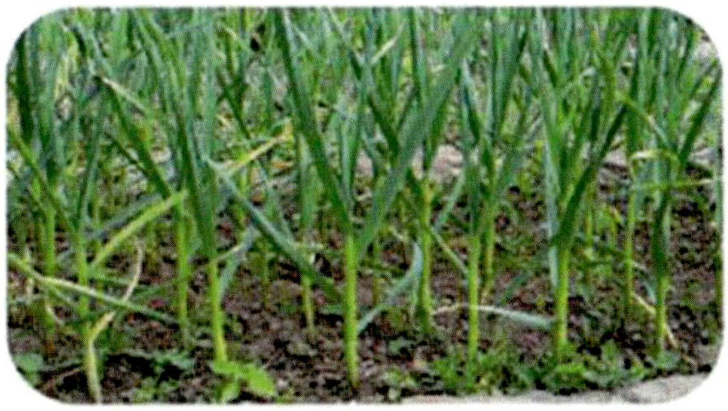

Garlic plant

Fig. (18). Garlic bulb and plant.

Scientific evidence has demonstrated that both garlic and its components possess preventive properties against common viral infections in humans by enhancing the immune system's response. The antibacterial qualities of garlic are attributed to allicin, which interacts with enzymes containing thiols, such as cysteine protease and alcohol dehydrogenases. These enzymes are vital for bacterial nutrition and metabolism [165].

1.3.16. Ginger

Ginger (*Zingiber officinale*) is a widely used spice in many Asian countries, belonging to the *Zingiberaceae* family (Fig. **19**). It is a slender, perennial upright herb characterized by a thick underground stem, or rhizome, from which the aerial stems grow up to approximately 1 meter tall and are entirely covered by leaf sheaths [166]. Chemical analysis of ginger oil reveals the presence of various compounds such as alkaloids, carbohydrates, glycosides, proteins, saponins, steroids, flavonoids, and terpenoids. Throughout history, this plant has been utilized in traditional medicine to address various ailments, including asthma, arthritis, stroke, toothache, paralysis, diabetes, and gastrointestinal issues [167]. The majority of components in ginger rhizomes consist of carbohydrates (50-70%), lipids (3-8%), terpenes, and phenolic substances. Among the terpene components found in ginger are zingiberene, bisabolene, farnesene, sesquiphellandrene, and curcumin, while phenolic substances include gingerol, paradols, and shogaol [168]. Notably, gingerols (23-25%) and shogaols (18-25%)

are more abundant compared to other types of compounds. Furthermore, ginger rhizomes contain minerals, phytosterols, vitamins (such as nicotinic acid and vitamin A), and amino acids. The aromatic components include zingiberene and bisabolene, while gingerols and shogaols contribute to the pungent taste and aroma [169]. Additionally, the ginger rhizome contains other related chemicals like 6-paradol, 1-dehydrogingerdione, 6- and 10-gingerdione, 4-, 6-, 8-, and 10-gingerdiol, and diarylheptanoids [170]. Ginger's distinct flavor and smell are attributed to volatile compounds such as shogaols and gingerols. Moreover, ginger exhibits valuable antibacterial properties and some antifungal effects. Active compounds in ginger help inhibit the growth of certain bacteria (*e.g.*, *E. coli, Proteus spp., Staphylococci, Streptococci, Salmonella*) in the colon *in vitro*, thus aiding in the control of flatulence caused by fermenting undigested carbohydrates. Ginger has also been found to inhibit the growth of *aspergillus*, a fungus that produces aflatoxin, a carcinogen [171]. Fresh ginger extract, or juice, has been observed to inhibit the growth of specific microorganisms, including *S. cerevisiae* (10%), *A. niger* (4%), *Mycoderma spp.* (12%), and *L. acidophilus* (14%) at room temperature [171]. Additionally, fresh ginger has shown dose-dependent inhibition of Human Respiratory Syncytial Virus (HRSV)-induced plaque formation in both HEp-2 and A549 cell lines. In contrast, dried ginger did not demonstrate dose-dependent inhibition [172]. A study conducted in Saudi Arabia noted that the consumption of ginger by COVID-19 patients increased from 36.2% before infection to 57.6% after infection. Interestingly, ginger users had a lower proportion of hospitalization for COVID-19 treatment (28.0%) compared to non-users (38.0%) [173].

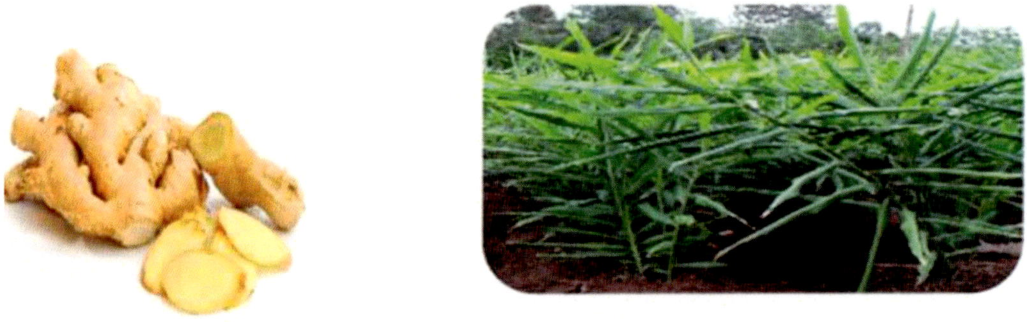

Fig. (19). Ginger rhizome and plant.

Mechanism: Several researchers have proposed that ginger contains phenolic compounds extracted using polar solvents and are primarily responsible for ginger's antimicrobial properties [174, 175]. These phenolic compounds act as denaturants for proteins, altering cell permeability and causing bacterial cells to swell and rupture. Furthermore, they are capable of chelating metal ions and binding to the active sites of metabolic enzymes or proteins, leading to a reduction in their activity and subsequently decreasing cell activity and reproduction. One particular ginger antifungal protein, known as SU2, has been isolated and shown to inhibit the mycelium formation of various fungi, such as *Botrytis cinerea, Fusarium oxysporum, Mycosphaerella arachidicola,* and *Physalospora piricola*. SU2 shares some similarities with the homeobox protein involved in fungal hyphal formation [176]. Fresh ginger alone has been found to effectively combat HRSV-induced plaque formation on airway epithelium by obstructing viral attachment and penetration into host cells through interactions with G and F proteins. In the lower respiratory system, fresh ginger may also prevent viral replication [172]. In a clinical trial, administering ginger extract to patients infected with the hepatitis C virus (HCV) resulted in reduced virus load, decreased levels of α-fetoprotein, and lowered levels of liver-related functional enzymes such as alanine aminotransferase and aspartate aminotransferase [177]. Molecular docking analyses have indicated that 6-gingerol, a compound found in ginger, exhibits a strong affinity for various virus proteins, including cathepsin K, the main protease, and SARS-CoV3C-like molecules, all of which are crucial for SARS-CoV-2 replication [178].

1.3.17. Sweet Neem

Murraya koenigii (L.) Spreng, commonly referred to as 'Curry Patta' or 'Meethi Neem,' originates from India (Fig. **20**). Its leaves are widely utilized to add flavor to various Indian dishes, including curries, chutneys, sambhar, and buttermilk, as well as preparations for egg, fish, and meat. These fresh leaves are rich in carotene, nicotinic acid, vitamin C, alkaloids, flavonoids, tannins, and volatile oil, and they have been reported to possess several beneficial properties like antioxidants, antibacterial, antifungal, anticarcinogenic, hypoglycemic, and antihypertensive activities [179]. The hypoglycemic characteristic of curry leaves is particularly noteworthy as it significantly reduces the body's blood sugar level. These leaves stimulate insulin production in the pancreas beta-cells upon consumption, leading to decreased starch breakdown into glucose, resulting in lower blood sugar levels. Moreover, curry leaves' high iron content effectively enhances hemoglobin and red blood cell count, acting as a natural blood purifier. This, in turn, alleviates symptoms of fatigue and tiredness and reduces the susceptibility to infections [180]. With its rich vitamin A and beta-carotene supply, curry leaves play a crucial role in promoting eye health and vision. They help prevent conditions like Xeropthalmia and night blindness by preventing corneal dryness and cloud formation in front of the eyes. Additionally, the potent antibacterial, antifungal, anti-inflammatory, and antioxidant qualities of curry leaves offer protection against various infections and microbes when consumed regularly [181]. Research on *M. koenigii* extracts has shown promising results in combating certain ailments. Ethanol extracts have demonstrated effectiveness against *Mycobacterium smegmatis*, particularly when compared to petroleum ether and water extracts. Additionally, the leaf extract exhibited cytotoxic and genotoxic effects and induced apoptosis in the mouse macrophage RAW 264.7 cell line [182]. Furthermore, the essential oil obtained from curry leaves showed potent inhibition against antibiotic-resistant bacteria such as *Staphylococcus aureus, Pseudomonas aeruginosa, Klebsiella pneumoniae, Escherichia coli,* and *Streptococcus pyogenes* [183, 184]. *Murraya koenigii* offers a multitude of health benefits and is a valuable addition to Indian cuisine, not only for its distinctive flavor but also for its potential medicinal properties.

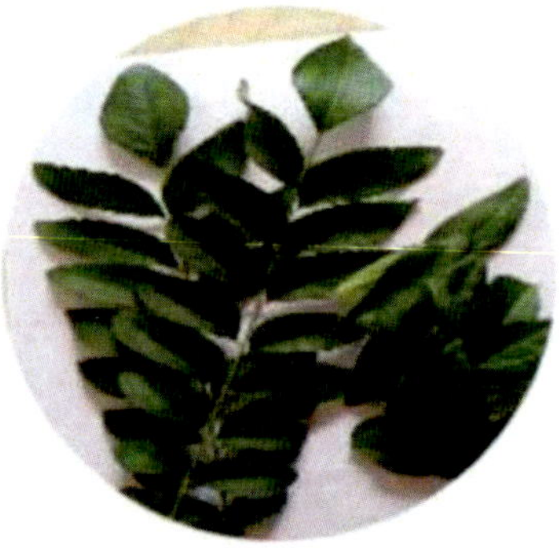

Sweet neem

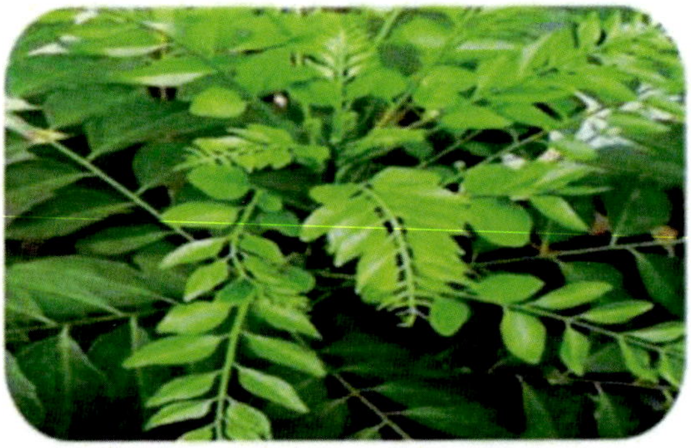

Sweet neem plant

Fig. (20). Sweet neem leaves and plant.

Mechanism: The fresh leaves of *Murraya koenigii* contain volatile oil, while the stem bark and roots have yielded Carbazole alkaloids and triterpene [183, 185]. A study demonstrated that *Murraya koenigii* extract increased the production of reactive oxygen species and nitric oxide, leading to enhanced intracellular killing of *M. smegmatis* in mouse macrophages [182]. Additionally, the administration of aqueous extract from both curry and olive leaves significantly lowered blood glucose levels in STZ-induced diabetic rats [186]. Curry leaves are abundant in polyphenols, terpenes, saponins, chlorophyll, and carotene. Saponins, known for their surfactant and detergent properties [187], can also contribute to the destruction of the coronavirus envelope by disrupting its lipid-based structure through foaming.

1.3.18. Star Anise

Illicium verum, a small to medium-sized evergreen tree belonging to the *Illiciaceae* genus, is the primary source of star anise (Fig. **21**). The Illicium genus comprises over 42 species and 166 variants, predominantly found in tropical regions of East Asia and Southeast Asia. There is significant variation in their morphology, habitat, and chemical composition. Among the various species in the Illicium genus, star anise (*Illicium verum*), Mexican anise (*Illicium mexicanum*), Japanese anise (*Illicium anisatum*), and star aniseed are the most popular. Star anise (*Illicium verum*) is the most well-known species [188]. It is cultivated for decorative purposes due to its attractive flowers, foliage, and aroma, resulting in numerous varieties. The plant is known by different names in various parts of the world, including star anise, bdiyn (Persian), phoolchakri (Hindi), badiane (French), and badian (Urdu) (English). Star anise is native to China and Vietnam, where it has been utilized for over three thousand years. The genus name "*Illicium*" is derived from the Latin word "alluring," signifying fragrance. In Southeast Asia, this evergreen tree called star anise can grow to heights of 12 to 16 feet [189]. The leaves are lanceolate, obovate-elliptic, and leathery, measuring 5–15 cm by 2–5 cm. The flowers are bisexual, axillary, or subterminal, measuring 1.5–4 cm in diameter and ranging from pink to dark crimson. The petals vary in number from seven to twelve and can have elliptic to ovate shapes. The fruit contains carpels that are 10 mm long, firm, wrinkled, and boat-shaped, each containing a seed. The fruit has a star-like appearance, reddish-brown in color, with six to eight whorls of follicles. The seeds are smooth, compact, brittle, and shiny brown [190]. Star anise is known for its rich content of ascorbic acid, protein, carbohydrates, and vitamin A. It also contains dietary fibers, sugars, and carbohydrates (65-75 g), as well as lipids (4-6 g) and proteins (2-4 g). Star anise is abundant in minerals such as salt, calcium, zinc, magnesium, potassium, iron, copper, and more. It provides approximately 359 Kcal of energy per 100 g. The distinct aroma of *Illicium verum* is attributed to the essential oil, which constitutes 2.5–3.5% of the fresh fruit and 8–9% of the dried material. The primary components of the volatile oil are trans-anethole and shikimic acid (3,4,5-trihydroxy-1-cyclohexene-1-carboxylic acid). Other chemical constituents found in star anise include sesquiterpenes, phenylpropanoids, lignans, flavonoids, and palmitic acid [191]. Due to its high concentration of trans-anethole, star anise oil possesses antiviral and cancer-preventive properties. It serves as a base for the production of various pharmaceutical products, including the anticonvulsant chloral. Star anise has also demonstrated significant antibacterial properties. Its main component, trans-anethole, exhibits antiviral, antibacterial, antifungal, and antiparasitic effects. Studies have shown that star anise inhibits the growth of *F. solani, F. graminearum,* and *F. oxysporum*, with complete inhibition observed at a 100 ppm dose [192]. Additionally, certain substances isolated from the roots of

Illicium verum, such as (-)-illicinoneA, 3,4-seco-(24Z)-cycloart-4(28), 24-diene-3,26-dioic acid, and 26-methyl ester, exhibit moderate anti-HIV activity [193]. The antiviral effects of star anise extracts have been observed against herpes simplex virus type 1, type 2, and bovine herpes virus type 1 [194 - 196]. *In-vitro* testing of three crude *Illicium verum* extracts—absolute methanol, 50% methanol, and aqueous extracts—has shown their ability to eliminate two Gram-positive bacteria (*Staphylococcus aureus* and *Listeria monocytogenes*), two Gram-negative bacteria (*Escherichia coli* and *Salmonella Arizona*), and two fungi (*Aspergillus fumigatus* and *Aspergillus niger*).

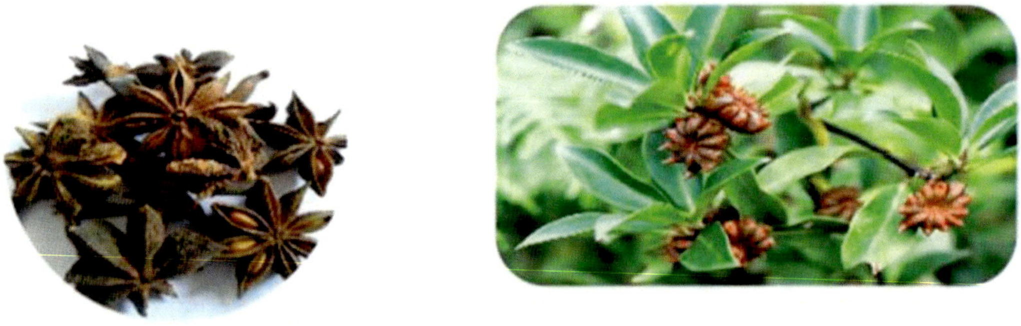

Star anise **Star anise plant**

Fig. (21). Star anise fruit and plant.

Mechanism: Several research studies have indicated that star anise possesses antibacterial properties, and this effect may arise from different mechanisms. Some studies suggest that it inhibits the synthesis of bacterial cell walls [198], while others propose that it accumulates in bacterial membranes, leading to energy depletion [199].

Additionally, star anise extract has been found to interfere with cell membrane permeability, resulting in increased permeability and the loss of cellular contents. This process can cause the disintegration of the cytoplasmic membrane and bring about structural and functional changes in cellular components, which can lead to mutations and damage to the cells [200]. Furthermore, star anise extracts have been shown to impede viral attachment to host cells and prevent their penetration [201].

Although the oil contains trans-anethole, which could potentially be transformed into natural fungicides [201] to hinder spore development in fungi [202], both the essential oil and trans-anethole exhibit strong inhibitory effects against all tested fungi.

1.3.19. Turmeric

Curcumin, a yellow polyphenolic compound sourced from the rhizome of *Curcuma longa L.* (turmeric) (Fig. **22**), has a long history of utilization in culinary and food coloring applications. Additionally, it has been employed in various medicinal preparations, playing a prominent role in Ayurveda and Chinese medicine [203]. Turmeric, a perennial plant from the *Zingiberaceae* family, is native to Southeast Asia and is well-known for its oblong leaves and brownish-yellow branched rhizomes [204]. It is extensively used in Asian countries such as China, Bangladesh, and Southeast Asia, serving as a food additive, preservative, and coloring agent. India is the leading producer, consumer, and exporter of turmeric, accounting for approximately 78 percent of global production. The significance of turmeric extends beyond its practical applications; it holds religious importance and is part of various rituals. In ancient Hindu medicine, turmeric was widely used to treat injuries, sprains, and swelling. Presently, traditional Indian medicine employs turmeric powder to address various ailments like biliary disorders, anorexia, cough, diabetes, hepatic disorders, rheumatism, sinusitis, and more. Turmeric, also referred to as "Haridra" or "Haldi," comprises essential components such as moisture, protein, fat, minerals, and carbohydrates. Steam distillation of its rhizomes yields an essential oil with constituents like -phellandrene, sabiene, cineol, borneol, zingiberene, and sesquiterpenes [205]. The key bioactive compound in turmeric is curcumin, accompanied by two others, desmethoxycurcumin and bisdemethoxycurcumin. Curcumin is responsible for the vibrant yellow color of turmeric and is recognized for its therapeutic effects. Approximately two to five percent of turmeric is composed of curcumin. This compound was first extracted from turmeric in 1815, and its structure, diferuloylmethane, was identified in 1910. Throughout the Indian subcontinent, turmeric has been widely used for over 6000 years for medicinal, cosmetic, dyeing, and culinary purposes [206]. Turmeric, historically known for its medicinal properties, was once utilized as a remedy for jaundice, an aid to suppress appetite and aid digestion. In ancient Indian and Chinese medicine, it served as an anti-inflammatory agent to address a range of issues such as gas, colic, toothaches, chest pains, and menstrual difficulties. This versatile spice was also applied to alleviate stomach and liver problems, promote wound healing, lighten scars, and even as a cosmetic agent. Its anticancer effects are primarily attributed to the induction of apoptosis, making it potentially valuable in managing rheumatism, carcinogenesis, and conditions linked to oxidative stress. Additionally, its anti-inflammatory and antioxidant properties could be clinically employed. The list of therapeutic applications includes AIDS/HIV, anemia, cancer, diabetes, food poisoning, gallstones, and more. Turmeric is also believed to alleviate lactation issues, insanity, poisoning, diarrhea, and urinary difficulties [207]. Beyond its culinary use as a flavor enhancer, turmeric, affectionately called

"Kitchen Queen," has long been a household remedy in traditional medicine to address various ailments such as biliary disorders, anorexia, cough, diabetic wounds, hepatic disorders, rheumatism, sinusitis, and others. Scientific studies have unveiled a broad spectrum of biological actions associated with turmeric [208]. The various activities of turmeric encompass anti-inflammatory, antioxidant, carcinogenic, anti-mutagenic, anticoagulant, antifertility, anti-diabetic, antibacterial, antifungal, antiprotozoal, antiviral, anti-fibrotic, antivenin, antiulcer, hypotensive, and hypo-cholesteric properties [209]. Moreover, it effectively cleanses and nourishes the blood, resulting in radiant and healthy skin. The herb's anti-bacterial and antiseptic qualities make it highly beneficial for treating skin conditions such as eczema, acne, and skin cancers while also aiding in the prevention of premature aging. Additionally, turmeric finds application in cosmetics and sunscreens [210]. In research, the aqueous extract of *C. longa* rhizome displayed significant antibacterial activity against *S. epidermis* ATCC 12228, *S. aureus* ATCC 25923, *K. pneumoniae* ATCC 10031, and *E. coli* ATCC 25922, with minimum inhibitory concentration (MIC) values ranging from 4 to 16 g/L and minimum bactericidal concentration (MBC) values ranging from 16 to 32 g/L [211]. For the methanol extract of turmeric, the MIC values against *B. subtilis* and *S. aureus* were found to be 16 g/mL and 128 g/mL, respectively [212]. Moreover, the ethanol extract exhibited the highest antimicrobial activity, with a MIC value of 3.91 to 125, based on a study of hexane and ethanol turmeric extract and curcuminoids [213]. These curcuminoids were isolated from *C. longa* and contained 86.5% curcumin [113]. The hexane and methanol extracts of *C. longa* demonstrated antibacterial effects against 13 different bacteria, including *Vibrio harveyi, Vibrio alginolyticus, Vibrio vulnificus, Vibrio parahaemolyticus, Vibrio cholerae, Bacillus subtilis, B. cereus, Aeromonas hydrophila, Streptococcus agalactiae,* and *Staphylococcus*. Notably, the curcuminoids in the extracts exhibited inhibitory effects against eight bacteria, including *S. agalactiae,* and *S. intermedius, S. epidermidis, S. aureus, A. hydrophila, B. subtilis, B. cereus,* and *Ed. tarda*. The minimum inhibitory concentration (MIC) ranges for the hexane extract and curcuminoids were found to be 125 to 1000 ppt and 3.91 to 500 ppt, respectively [113]. Additionally, curcumin showed effectiveness against methicillin-resistant *S. aureus* (MRSA) bacteria, with MIC values ranging from 125-250 g/mL. Studies have indicated that curcumin and its bioconjugates are highly effective against various viruses, including Vesicular stomatitis virus (VSV), herpes simplex virus (HSV), flock house virus (FHV), respiratory syncytial virus (RSV), parainfluenza virus type 3 (PIV-3), and feline infectious peritonitis virus (FIPV) [214, 215]. Notably, clinical research has shown promising results of nano-encapsulated curcumin in COVID-19 patients, with those receiving nano-curcumin experiencing a significant reduction in clinical symptoms such as fever, cough, and dyspnea [216, 217].

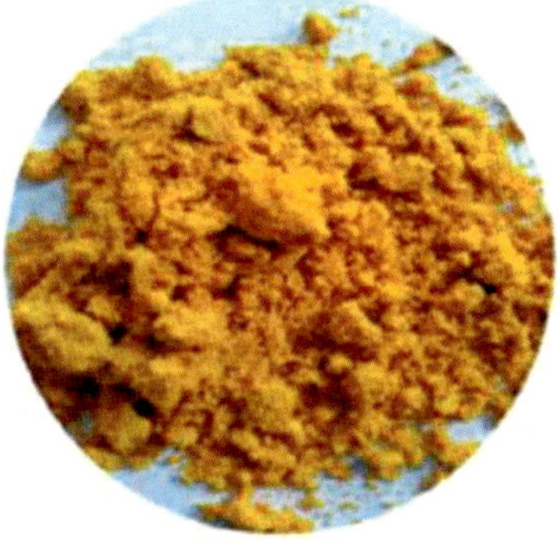

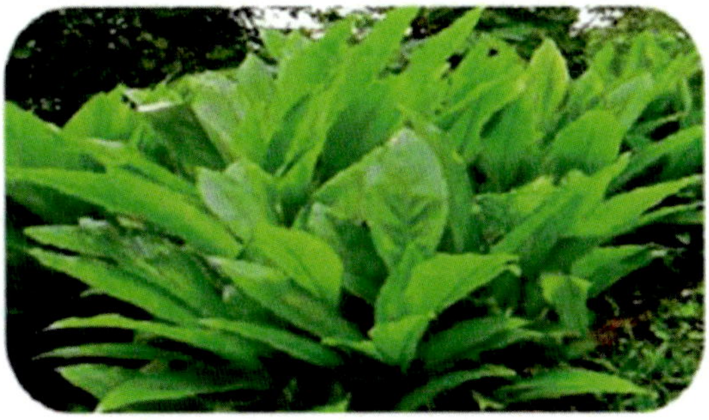

Turmuric powder **Turmuric plant**

Fig. (22). Turmeric powder and plant.

Mechanism: One research study confirmed that curcumin exhibits significantly higher sensitivity to Gram-positive bacteria compared to Gram-negative bacteria. Additionally, there have been reports about curcumin's antibiofilm properties against various bacterial species [218]. Curcumin acts by inhibiting bacterial DNA replication and modulating gene expression. Moreover, it disrupts the bacterial cell membrane and impairs the motility of microorganisms [219]. Curcumin also shows anti-adhesive effects at sub-inhibitory concentrations, hindering *C. albicans* biofilm formation.

Furthermore, curcumin demonstrates a broad spectrum of antiviral activity, effectively targeting multiple viruses [219]. The enzyme inosine monophosphate dehydrogenase (IMPDH), which plays a vital role in the production of guanine nucleotides, has been identified as a potential therapeutic target for antiviral and anticancer drugs [184]. IMPDH is responsible for catalyzing the oxidation of several purines, which is essential for DNA and RNA synthesis, as well as signal transduction. By interfering with this enzyme's functioning, Curcumin has been highlighted as a promising antiviral agent [219].

CONCLUSION

Common Indian spices are outlined with reference to their antimicrobial, antibacterial, and antifungal activity. The majority of Indian spices have demonstrated significant activities against pathogens. In order to increase food safety and shelf life, lower the danger of food poisoning and spoilage, and treat some infectious diseases, these spices may be employed. All of these have historically been employed in traditional medicines and are now employed in alternative healthcare. Indian culinary products almost always contain spice or a well-chosen blend of spices. Furthermore, because spices are easily accessible in the home, elite, underprivileged, and aboriginal populations use them for sporadic medical requirements. However, only a few numbers of spices are used specifically for diseases with a systematic methodology. These Indian spices include a variety of essential oils and/or aromatic chemicals as prime constituents and secondary metabolites. Due to the antibacterial and antifungal properties of their natural constituents, spices can impact both human illnesses (food safety) and food spoilage microorganisms (food preservation) during the food preparation process. As it has been shown that the combinations of several spices have more inhibitory effects on certain bacteria than those of individual spices, the interactions of additional spices should be explored and evaluated in the future to suppress diverse microorganisms in various food products.

Because the pharmaceutical industry has been committed to producing novel therapies for a variety of health conditions and producing new or improved molecules working against spoilage bacteria, researchers can draw inspiration from the study of spices, natural chemicals, and cutting-edge combination technologies. The American Food and Drug Administration (US FDA) has deemed spices generally safe when made from natural herbs and plants. Their organoleptic characteristics may significantly impact the outcomes of *In-vitro* and *In-vivo* research. Since they can be used with or without other technologies, mixtures of spices or their pure natural constituents offer a possible solution to this issue.

REFERENCES

[1] Rathore MS, Shekhawat NS. Incredible spices of India: from traditions to cuisine. Am-Eurasian J Bot 2008; 1(3): 85-9. Corpus ID: 73923659.

[2] Jiang TA. Health Benefits of Culinary Herbs and Spices. J AOAC Int 2019; 102(2): 395-411. [http://dx.doi.org/10.5740/jaoacint.18-0418] [PMID: 30651162]

[3] Aafreen MM, Geetha RV, Thangavelu L. Evaluation of anti-inflammatory action of Laurus nobilis-an *in vitro* study. Int J Res Pharm 2019; 1209-13. [http://dx.doi.org/10.26452/IJRPS.V10I2.408]

[4] Sainani GS, Desai DB, Gorhe NH, Natu SM, Pise DV, Sainani PG. Effect of dietary garlic and onion on serum lipid profile in Jain community. Indian J Med Res 1979; 69: 776-80. [PMID: 511261]

[5] Thatte UM, Dahanukar SA. Ayurveda and contemporary scientific thought. Trends Pharmacol Sci 1986; 7: 247-51. [http://dx.doi.org/10.1016/0165-6147(86)90336-6]

[6] Ma L, Yao L. Antiviral effects of plant-derived essential oils and their components: an updated review. Molecules 2020; 25(11): 2627. [http://dx.doi.org/10.3390/molecules25112627] [PMID: 32516954]

[7] Singh NA, Kumar P, Jyoti , Kumar N. Spices and herbs: Potential antiviral preventives and immunity boosters during COVID-19. Phytother Res 2021; 35(5): 2745-57. [http://dx.doi.org/10.1002/ptr.7019] [PMID: 33511704]

[8] Li S, Yuan W, Deng G, Wang P, Yang P, Aggarwal B. Chemical composition and product quality

control of turmeric (*Curcuma longa* L.). Pharm Crop 2011; 5(1): 28-54.
[http://dx.doi.org/10.2174/2210290601102010028]

[9] Augustine A, Anitha P, Sreerag G, Sreeraj G. Biological activities of curcuminoids, other biomolecules from turmeric and their derivatives – A review. J Trad Comp Med 2017; 7(2): 205-33.
[http://dx.doi.org/10.1016/j.jtcme.2016.05.005]

[10] Shan B, Cai YZ, Brooks JD, Corke H. Antibacterial and antioxidant effects of five spice and herb extracts as natural preservatives of raw pork. J Sci Food Agric 2009; 89(11): 1879-85.
[http://dx.doi.org/10.1002/jsfa.3667]

[11] Chaieb K, Hajlaoui H, Zmantar T. The chemical composition and biological activity of clove essential oil, Eugenia caryophyllata (Syzigium aromaticum L. Myrtaceae): a short review. Phyto Res 2007; 21(6): 501-6.
[http://dx.doi.org/10.1002/ptr.2124]

[12] Deepa G, Ayesha S, Nishtha K, Thankamani M. Comparative evaluation of various total antioxidant capacity assays applied to phytochemical compounds of Indian culinary spices. Int Food Res J 2013; 20(4): 221-7. Corpus ID: 67797144.

[13] Rahmatullah M, Noman A, Hossan MS, *et al.* A survey of medicinal plants in two areas of Dinajpur district, Bangladesh including plants which can be used as functional foods. Ame Euro J Sus Agri 2009; 3: 862-76. Corpus ID: 70365727.

[14] Shukla S, Mistry H, Patel V, Jogi B. Pharmacognostical, preliminary phytochemical studies and analgesic activity of *Amomum subulatum* Roxb. Pharma Sci Monitor 2010; 1: 90-102. Corpus ID: 42087158.

[15] Majdalawieh AF, Carr RI. *In vitro* investigation of the potential immunomodulatory and anti-cancer activities of black pepper (*Piper nigrum*) and cardamom (*Elettaria cardamomum*). J Med Food 2010; 13(2): 371-81.
[http://dx.doi.org/10.1089/jmf.2009.1131] [PMID: 20210607]

[16] Qian-Qian M, Xiao-Yu X, Shi-Yu C. Bioactive compounds and bioactivities of ginger. foods 2019; 8(6): 185.
[http://dx.doi.org/10.3390/foods8060185]

[17] Adib-Hajbaghery M, Hosseini FS. Investigating the effects of inhaling ginger essence on post-nephrectomy nausea and vomiting. Complement Ther Med 2015; 23(6): 827-31.
[http://dx.doi.org/10.1016/j.ctim.2015.10.002] [PMID: 26645524]

[18] Valiollah H, Naser A. Hypolipidemic activity of Anethum graveolens in rats. Phyto res 2019; 22(3): 372-5.
[http://dx.doi.org/10.1002/ptr.2329]

[19] Valadi A, Nasri S, Abbasi N, Amir GR. Antinociceptive and anti-inflammatory effects of hydroalcoholic extract from the seed of *Anethum graveolens* L. J Med Pla 2010; 9(34): 124-30.

[20] Naseri M, Mojab F, Khodadoost M, *et al.* The study of anti-inflammatory activity of oil-based dill (*Anethum graveolens* L.) extract used topically in formalin-induced inflammation male rat paw. Iran J Pharm Res 2012; 11(4): 1169-74.
[PMID: 24250550]

[21] Sayyah M, Valizadeh J, Kamalinejad M. Anticonvulsant activity of the leaf essential oil of *Laurus nobilis* against pentylenetetrazole- and maximal electroshock-induced seizures. Phytomedicine 2002; 9(3): 212-6.
[http://dx.doi.org/10.1078/0944-7113-00113] [PMID: 12046861]

[22] Jayaprakasha GK, Rao LJM. Chemistry, biogenesis, and biological activities of *Cinnamomum zeylanicum.* Crit Rev Food Sci Nutr 2011; 51(6): 547-62.
[http://dx.doi.org/10.1080/10408391003699550] [PMID: 21929331]

[23] Bellamy DA, Pfister A. Spices overview World medicine: plants, patients and people. Oxford:

Blackwell Publishers 1992.

[24] Ramaswamy S, Sengottuvelu S, Sherief SH, *et al.* Gastroprotective activity of ethanolic extract of *Trachyspermum ammi* fruit. Int J Pharm Biol Sci 2010; 1: 1-15. Corpus ID: 12593438

[25] Platel K, Srinivasan K. Studies on the influence of dietary spices on food transit time in experimental rats. Nutr Res 2001; 21(9): 1309-14. [http://dx.doi.org/10.1016/S0271-5317(01)00331-1]

[26] Walsh SE, Maillard JY, Russell AD, Catrenich CE, Charbonneau DL, Bartolo RG. Activity and mechanisms of action of selected biocidal agents on Gram-positive and -negative bacteria. J Appl Microbiol 2003; 94(2): 240-7. [http://dx.doi.org/10.1046/j.1365-2672.2003.01825.x] [PMID: 12534815]

[27] Nuñez L, D' Aquino M, D'aquinobrazilian M. Microbicide activity of clove essential oil (Eugenia caryophyllata). Braz J Microbiol 2012; 43(4): 1255-60. [http://dx.doi.org/10.1590/S1517-83822012000400003] [PMID: 24031950]

[28] Nzeako BC, Al-Kharousi ZS, Al-Mahrooqui Z. Antimicrobial activities of clove and thyme extracts. Sultan Qaboos Univ Med J 2006; 6(1): 33-9. [PMID: 21748125]

[29] Benencia F, Courrèges MC. *In vitro* and *in vivo* activity of eugenol on human herpesvirus. Phytother Res 2000; 14(7): 495-500. [http://dx.doi.org/10.1002/1099-1573(200011)14:7<495::AID-PTR650>3.0.CO;2-8] [PMID: 11054837]

[30] Yadav MK, Park SW, Chae SW, Song JJ, Kim HC. Antimicrobial activities of *Eugenia caryophyllata* extract and its major chemical constituent eugenol against *Streptococcus pneumoniae*. Acta Pathol Microbiol Scand Suppl 2013; 121(12): 1198-206. [http://dx.doi.org/10.1111/apm.12067] [PMID: 23594212]

[31] Baskaran SA, Kollanoor-Johny A, Nair MS, Venkitanarayanan K. Efficacy of plant-derived antimicrobials in controlling enterohemorrhagic *Escherichia coli* virulence *in vitro.* J Food Prot 2016; 79(11): 1965-70. [http://dx.doi.org/10.4315/0362-028X.JFP-16-104] [PMID: 28221905]

[32] Ajiboye TO, Mohammed AO, Bello SA, *et al.* Antibacterial activity of *Syzygium aromaticum* seed: Studies on oxidative stress biomarkers and membrane permeability. Microb Pathog 2016; 95: 208-15. [http://dx.doi.org/10.1016/j.micpath.2016.03.011] [PMID: 27038843]

[33] Ribeiro-Santos R, Andrade M, Madella D, *et al.* Revisiting an ancient spice with medicinal purposes: Cinnamon. Trends Food Sci Technol 2017; 62: 154-69. [http://dx.doi.org/10.1016/j.tifs.2017.02.011]

[34] Pathirana HNKS, Wimalasena SHMP, De Silva BCJ, Hossain S, Heo GJ. Antibacterial activity of cinnamon (*Cinnamomum zeylanicum*) essential oil and cinnamaldehyde against fish pathogenic bacteria isolated from cultured olive flounder *Paralichthys olivaceus.* Indian J Fish 2019; 66(2): 86-92. [http://dx.doi.org/10.21077/ijf.2019.66.2.85023-12]

[35] El Atki Y, Aouam I, El Kamari F, *et al.* Antibacterial activity of cinnamon essential oils and their synergistic potential with antibiotics. J Adv Pharm Technol Res 2019; 10(2): 63-7. [http://dx.doi.org/10.4103/japtr.JAPTR_366_18] [PMID: 31041184]

[36] Utchariyakiat I, Surassmo S, Jaturanpinyo M, Khuntayaporn P, Chomnawang MT. Efficacy of cinnamon bark oil and cinnamaldehyde on anti-multidrug resistant *Pseudomonas aeruginosa* and the synergistic effects in combination with other antimicrobial agents. BMC Complement Altern Med 2016; 16(1): 158. [http://dx.doi.org/10.1186/s12906-016-1134-9] [PMID: 27245046]

[37] Astani A, Reichling J, Schnitzler P. Comparative study on the antiviral activity of selected monoterpenes derived from essential oils. Phytother Res 2010; 24(5): 673-9.

[http://dx.doi.org/10.1002/ptr.2955] [PMID: 19653195]

[38] Vimalanathan S, Hudson J. Anti-influenza virus activity of essential oils and vapors. Am J Essent 2014; 2: 47-53. Corpus ID: 19456298.

[39] Shreaz S, Bhatia R, Khan N, *et al.* Spice oil cinnamaldehyde exhibits potent anticandidal activity against fluconazole resistant clinical isolates. Fitoterapia 2011; 82(7): 1012-20. [http://dx.doi.org/10.1016/j.fitote.2011.06.004] [PMID: 21708228]

[40] Huang H, Wang Y. The protective effect of cinnamaldehyde on lipopolysaccharide induced acute lung injury in mice. Cell Mol Biol 2017; 63(8): 58-63. [http://dx.doi.org/10.14715/cmb/2017.63.8.13] [PMID: 28886315]

[41] Bouhdid S, Abrini J, Amensour M, Zhiri A, Espuny MJ, Manresa A. Functional and ultrastructural changes in *Pseudomonas aeruginosa* and *Staphylococcus aureus* cells induced by *Cinnamomum verum* essential oil. J Appl Microbiol 2010; 109(4): 1139-49. [http://dx.doi.org/10.1111/j.1365-2672.2010.04740.x] [PMID: 20456525]

[42] Ma YH, Deng JH, Wang GS, Zhang XG, Wang AX, Si RL. Therapeutic effect of cinnamon oil on gastric candida albicans infection in mice. World Chin J Digestology 2009; 17(15): 1545-7. [http://dx.doi.org/10.11569/wcjd.v17.i15.1545]

[43] Xie XM, Xu Y. Advances in study on anti-fungal mechanism of Chinese herbal medicines. Zhongguo Zhongyao Zazhi 2004; 29(3): 200-2. [PMID: 15706838]

[44] Sharma S, Sharma J, Kaur G. Therapeutic uses of *Elettaria cardamomum.* Int J Drug Form Res 2011; 2: 102-8.

[45] Savan EK, Kucukbay FZ. Essential oil composition of *Elettaria cardamomum* Maton. J Appl Biosci 2013; 7: 42-5. Corpus ID: 98407949.

[46] Abdullah AA, Asghar A, Butt MS, Shahid M, Huang Q. Evaluating the antimicrobial potential of green cardamom essential oil focusing on quorum sensing inhibition of *Chromobacterium violaceum.* J Food Sci Technol 2017; 54(8): 2306-15. [http://dx.doi.org/10.1007/s13197-017-2668-7] [PMID: 28740287]

[47] de Sousa JP, Torres RA, de Azerêdo GA, Figueiredo RCBQ, Vasconcelos MAS, de Souza EL. Carvacrol and 1,8-cineole alone or in combination at sublethal concentrations induce changes in the cell morphology and membrane permeability of *Pseudomonas fluorescens* in a vegetable-based broth. Int J Food Microbiol 2012; 158(1): 9-13. [http://dx.doi.org/10.1016/j.ijfoodmicro.2012.06.008] [PMID: 22795513]

[48] Brewer MS. Natural antioxidants: sources, compounds, mechanisms of action, and potential applications. Compr Rev Food Sci Food Saf 2011; 10(4): 221-47. [http://dx.doi.org/10.1111/j.1541-4337.2011.00156.x]

[49] Bhaswant M, Poudyal H, Mathai M, Ward L, Mouatt P, Brown L. Green and black cardamom in a diet-induced rat model of metabolic syndrome. Nutrients 2015; 7(9): 7691-707. [http://dx.doi.org/10.3390/nu7095360] [PMID: 26378573]

[50] Abdallah EM, Abdalla WE. Black pepper fruit (*Piper nigrum* L.) as antibacterial agent: A mini-review. J Bacteriol Mycol 2018; 6(2): 141-5. [http://dx.doi.org/10.15406/jbmoa.2018.06.00192]

[51] Pradhan KJ, Variya PS, Bandeka JR. Antimicrobial activity of novel phenolic compounds from green pepper (*Piper nigrum* L.). J Food. Sci Tech (Paris) 1999; 32: 121-3. [http://dx.doi.org/10.1006/fstl.1998.0508]

[52] Shiva Rani SK, Saxena N. Antimicrobial Activity of Black Pepper (*Piper nigrum* L.). Glob J Pharmacol 2013; 7(1): 87-90. [http://dx.doi.org/10.5829/idosi.gjp.2013.7.1.1104]

[53] Priya NC, Saravana Kumari P. Activities and Cytotoxicity Assay of Seed Extracts of *Piper longum* and *Piper nigrum* on Human Cell Lines. Int J Pharm Sci Rev Res 2017; 44(1): 197-202.

[54] Rout J, Swain BC, Tripathy U. *In silico* investigation of spice molecules as potent inhibitor of SARS-CoV-2. J Biomol Struct Dyn 2020; 2: 1-15.
[PMID: 32938313]

[55] Nag A, Chowdhury RR. Piperine, an alkaloid of black pepper seeds can effectively inhibit the antiviral enzymes of Dengue and Ebola viruses, an *in silico* molecular docking study. Virusdisease 2020; 31(3): 308-15.
[http://dx.doi.org/10.1007/s13337-020-00619-6] [PMID: 32904842]

[56] Lin LT, Hsu WC, Lin CC. Antiviral natural products and herbal medicines. J Tradit Complement Med 2014; 4(1): 24-35.
[http://dx.doi.org/10.4103/2225-4110.124335] [PMID: 24872930]

[57] Sharma RP, Singh RS, Verma TP, Tailor BL, Sharma SS, Singh SK. Coriander the Taste of Vegetables: Present and Future Prospectus for Coriander Seed Production in Southeast Rajasthan. Econ Aff 2014; 59(3): 345-54.
[http://dx.doi.org/10.5958/0976-4666.2014.00003.5]

[58] Anwar F, Sulman M, Hussain AI, Saari N, Iqbal S. Physicochemical composition of hydro-distilled essential oil from coriander (*Coriandrum sativum* L.) seeds cultivated in Pakistan. J Med Plants Res 2011; 5: 3537-44.
[http://dx.doi.org/10.5897/JMPR.9000978]

[59] Nejad Ebrahimi S, Hadian J, Ranjbar H. Essential oil compositions of different accessions of *Coriandrum sativum* L. from Iran. Nat Prod Res 2010; 24(14): 1287-94.
[http://dx.doi.org/10.1080/14786410903132316] [PMID: 20803372]

[60] Msaada K, Taarit MB, Hosni K, Hammami M, Marzouk B. Regional and maturational effects on essential oils yields and composition of coriander (*Coriandrum sativum* L.) fruits. Sci Hortic (Amsterdam) 2009; 122(1): 116-24.
[http://dx.doi.org/10.1016/j.scienta.2009.04.008]

[61] Filomena Silva F, Domingues FC. Antimicrobial activity of coriander oil and its effectiveness as food preservative. Crit Rev Food Sci Nut 2017; 57(1): 35-47.
[http://dx.doi.org/10.1080/10408398.2013.847818]

[62] Silva F, Ferreira S, Queiroz JA, Domingues FC. Coriander (Coriandrum sativum L.) essential oil: its antibacterial activity and mode of action evaluated by flow cytometry. J Med Microbiol 2011; 60(10): 1479-86.
[http://dx.doi.org/10.1099/jmm.0.034157-0] [PMID: 21862758]

[63] Silva F, Ferreira S, Duarte A, Mendonça DI, Domingues FC. Antifungal activity of *Coriandrum sativum* essential oil, its mode of action against Candida species and potential synergism with amphotericin B. Phytomedicine 2011; 19(1): 42-7.
[http://dx.doi.org/10.1016/j.phymed.2011.06.033] [PMID: 21788125]

[64] Roby MHH, Sarhan MA, Selim KAH, Khalel KI. Antioxidant and antimicrobial activities of essential oil and extracts of fennel (Foeniculum vulgare L.) and chamomile (Matricaria chamomilla L.). Ind Crops Prod 2013; 44: 437-45.
[http://dx.doi.org/10.1016/j.indcrop.2012.10.012]

[65] Díaz-Maroto MC, Pérez-Coello MS, Esteban J, Sanz J. Comparison of the volatile composition of wild fennel samples (*Foeniculum vulgare* Mill.) from central Spain. J Agric Food Chem 2006; 54(18): 6814-8.
[http://dx.doi.org/10.1021/jf0609532] [PMID: 16939344]

[66] Choi EM, Hwang JK. Antiinflammatory, analgesic and antioxidant activities of the fruit of *Foeniculum vulgare*. Fitoterapia 2004; 75(6): 557-65.

[http://dx.doi.org/10.1016/j.fitote.2004.05.005] [PMID: 15351109]

[67] Gulfraz M, Mehmood S, Minhas N, *et al.* Composition and antimicrobial properties of essential oil of *Foeniculum vulgare.* Afr J Biotechnol 2008; 7(24): 4364-8.

[68] Orhan İE, Özçelik B, Kartal M, Kan Y. Antimicrobial and antiviral effects of essential oils from selected Umbelliferae and Labiatae plants and individual essential oil components. Turk J Biol 2012; 36(3): 239-46.
[http://dx.doi.org/10.3906/biy-0912-30]

[69] Park SH, Seong I. Antifungal effects of the extracts and essential oils from *Foeniculum vulgare* and *Illicium verum* against *Candida albicans.* Korean J Med Mycol 2010; 15(4): 157-64.

[70] Thakur N, Sareen N, Shama B, Jagota K. Studies on *in vitro* antifungal activity of *Foeniculum vulgare* Mill. against spoilage fungi. GJBB 2013; 2(3): 427-30. Corpus ID: 29120118

[71] Samah AA, Bahaeldin KE, Afra AAB, Aisha ZA. *In Vitro* Test of Antimicrobial Activity of *Foeniculum Vulgare* Mill. (Fennel) Essential Oil. J Multidiscip Eng Sci Stud 2017; 3(4): 1609-14.

[72] Diao WR, Hu QP, Zhang H, Xu JG. Chemical composition, antibacterial activity and mechanism of action of essential oil from seeds of fennel (Foeniculum vulgare Mill.). Food Control 2014; 35(1): 109-16.
[http://dx.doi.org/10.1016/j.foodcont.2013.06.056]

[73] Zeng H, Chen X, Liang J. *In vitro* antifungal activity and mechanism of essential oil from fennel (*Foeniculum vulgare* L.) on dermatophyte species. J Med Microbiol 2015; 64(1): 93-103.
[http://dx.doi.org/10.1099/jmm.0.077768-0] [PMID: 25351709]

[74] Astani A, Reichling J, Schnitzler P. Screening for antiviral activities of isolated compounds from essential oils. Evid Based Complement Alternat Med 2011; 2011: 1-8.
[http://dx.doi.org/10.1093/ecam/nep187] [PMID: 20008902]

[75] Wanner J, Bail S, Jirovetz L, *et al.* Chemical composition and antimicrobial activity of cumin oil (*Cuminum cyminum*, Apiaceae). Nat Prod Commun 2010; 5(9): 1934578X1000500.
[http://dx.doi.org/10.1177/1934578X1000500904] [PMID: 20922990]

[76] Mageed MAAE, Mansour AF, El Massry KF, Ramadan MM, Shaheen MS, Shaaban H. Effect of microwaves on essential oils of coriander and cumin seeds and on their antioxidant and antimicrobial activities. J Essent Oil-Bear Plants 2012; 15(4): 614-27.
[http://dx.doi.org/10.1080/0972060X.2012.10644096]

[77] Sheikh MI, Islam S, Rahman A, *et al.* Control of Some Human Pathogenic Bacteria by Seed Extracts of Cumin (*Cuminum cyminum* L.). ACS Agric Conspec Sci 2010; 75(1): 39-44. Corpus ID: 37790380.

[78] Mohamadein MM, Farrag RM, Mekawey AAI. Antiviral and Antidermatophytic Activity of a Compound Extracted from *Cuminum cyminum* Seeds. Biomed Pharmacol J 2015; 8(2): 573-80.
[http://dx.doi.org/10.13005/bpj/800]

[79] Motamedifar M, Ghafari N, Talezadeh Shirazi P. The Effect of Cumin Seed Extracts against *Herpes Simplex* Virus Type 1 in Vero Cell Culture. Iran J Basic Med Sci 2010; 35(4): 304-9. Corpus ID: 55097392.

[80] Wongkattiya N, Sanguansermsri P, Fraser IH, Sanguansermsri D. Antibacterial activity of cuminaldehyde on food-borne pathogens, the bioactive component of essential oil from *Cuminum cyminum* L. collected in Thailand. J Complement Integr Med 2019; 16(4): 20180195.
[http://dx.doi.org/10.1515/jcim-2018-0195] [PMID: 31129652]

[81] Shekhawat GS, Jana S. *Anethum graveolens*: An Indian traditional medicinal herb and spice. Pharmacogn Rev 2010; 4(8): 179-84.
[http://dx.doi.org/10.4103/0973-7847.70915] [PMID: 22228959]

[82] Blank I, Grosch W. Evaluation of potent odorants in dill seed and dill herb (*Anethum graveolens* L.) by aroma extract dilution analysis. J Food Sci 1991; 56(1): 63-7.

[http://dx.doi.org/10.1111/j.1365-2621.1991.tb07976.x]

[83] Huopalahti R, Linko RR. Composition and content of aroma compounds in dill, *Anethum graveolens* L., at three different growth stages. J Agric Food Chem 1983; 31(2): 331-3. [http://dx.doi.org/10.1021/jf00116a036]

[84] Pulliah T, Ed. Medicinal Plants in Indiai: Regency Publications New Delhi 2002, pp. 55-56.

[85] Jirovetz L, Buchbauer G, Stoyanova AS, Georgiev EV, Damianova ST. Composition, quality control, and antimicrobial activity of the essential oil of long-time stored dill (Anethum graveolens L.) seeds from Bulgaria. J Agric Food Chem 2003; 51(13): 3854-7. [http://dx.doi.org/10.1021/jf030004y] [PMID: 12797755]

[86] López P, Sánchez C, Batlle R, Nerín C. Solid- and vapor-phase antimicrobial activities of six essential oils: susceptibility of selected foodborne bacterial and fungal strains. J Agric Food Chem 2005; 53(17): 6939-46. [http://dx.doi.org/10.1021/jf050709v] [PMID: 16104824]

[87] Derakhshan S, Navidinia M, Ahmadi A. Antibacterial activity of dill (Anethum graveolens) essential oil and antibiofilm activity of cumin (Cuminum cyminum) Alcoholic Extract. Infect Epidemiol Microb 2017; 3(4): 122-6. [http://dx.doi.org/10.18869/MODARES.IEM.3.4.122]

[88] Badr AN, Nada F, Shehata MG, Amra HA. Anti-mycotic and anti-mycotoxigenic properties of Egyptian dill. J Appl Sci (Faisalabad) 2017; 17(4): 184-95. [http://dx.doi.org/10.3923/jas.2017.184.195]

[89] Burt S. Essential oils: their antibacterial properties and potential applications in foods—a review. Int J Food Microbiol 2004; 94(3): 223-53. [http://dx.doi.org/10.1016/j.ijfoodmicro.2004.03.022] [PMID: 15246235]

[90] Sikkema J, de Bont JA, Poolman B. Mechanisms of membrane toxicity of hydrocarbons. Microbiol Rev 1995; 59(2): 201-22. [http://dx.doi.org/10.1128/mr.59.2.201-222.1995] [PMID: 7603409]

[91] Conner DE, Beuchat LR. Effects of essential oils from plants on growth of food spoilage yeasts. J Food Sci 1984; 49(2): 429-34. [http://dx.doi.org/10.1111/j.1365-2621.1984.tb12437.x]

[92] Conner DE, Beuchat LR. Sensitivity of heat-stressed yeasts to essential oils of plants. Appl Environ Microbiol 1984; 47(2): 229-33. [http://dx.doi.org/10.1128/aem.47.2.229-233.1984] [PMID: 6712207]

[93] Nychas GJ. Natural Antimicrobial from Plants.New Methods of Food Preservation. Glasgow: Blackie Academic and Professional 1995; pp. 59-89. [http://dx.doi.org/10.1007/978-1-4615-2105-1_4]

[94] Helal GA, Sarhan MM, Abu Shahla ANK, Abou El-Khair EK. Effects of*Cymbopogon citratus* L. essential oil on the growth, morphogenesis and aflatoxin production of*Aspergillus flavus* ML2-strain. J Basic Microbiol 2007; 47(1): 5-15. [http://dx.doi.org/10.1002/jobm.200610137] [PMID: 17304618]

[95] Rasooli I, Owlia P. Chemoprevention by thyme oils of *Aspergillus parasiticus* growth and aflatoxin production. Phytochemistry 2005; 66(24): 2851-6. [http://dx.doi.org/10.1016/j.phytochem.2005.09.029] [PMID: 16289146]

[96] Singh V, Amdekar S, Verma O. *Ocimum sanctum* (tulsi): Biopharmacological Activities. Webmed Central Pharmacol 2010; 1(10): 1-7.

[97] Chiang LC, Ng LT, Cheng PW, Chiang W, Lin CC. Antiviral activities of extracts and selected pure constituents of *Ocimum basilicum*. Clin Exp Pharmacol Physiol 2005; 32(10): 811-6. [http://dx.doi.org/10.1111/j.1440-1681.2005.04270.x] [PMID: 16173941]

[98] Mallikarjun S, Rao A, Rajesh G, Shenoy R, Pai M. Antimicrobial efficacy of Tulsi leaf (*Ocimum sanctum*) extract on periodontal pathogens: An *in vitro* study. J Indian Soc Periodontol 2016; 20(2): 145-50.
[PMID: 27143825]

[99] Yamani HA, Pang EC, Mantri N, Deighton MA. Antimicrobial Activity of Tulsi (*Ocimum tenuiflorum*) Essential Oil and Their Major Constituents against Three Species of Bacteria. Front Microbiol 2016; 7: 681.
[http://dx.doi.org/10.3389/fmicb.2016.00681] [PMID: 27242708]

[100] Singh S, Malhotra M, Majumdar DK. Antibacterial activity of *Ocimum sanctum* L. fixed oil. Indian J Exp Biol 2005; 43(9): 835-7.
[PMID: 16187537]

[101] Geeta , Vasudevan DM, Kedlaya R, Deepa S, Ballal M. Activity of Ocimum sanctum (the traditional Indian medicinal plant) against the enteric pathogens. Indian J Med Sci 2001; 55(8): 434-438, 472.
[PMID: 12026506]

[102] Novotný L, Vachálková A, Biggs D. Ursolic acid: an anti-tumorigenic and chemopreventive activity. Minireview. Neoplasma 2001; 48(4): 241-6.
[PMID: 11712672]

[103] Jamshidi N, Cohen MM. The clinical efficacy and safety of Tulsi in humans: A systematic review of the literature. Evid Based Complement Alternat Med 2017; 2017: 1-13.
[http://dx.doi.org/10.1155/2017/9217567] [PMID: 28400848]

[104] Pattanayak P, Behera P, Das D, Panda S. *Ocimum sanctum* Linn. A reservoir plant for therapeutic applications: An overview. Pharmacogn Rev 2010; 4(7): 95-105.
[http://dx.doi.org/10.4103/0973-7847.65323] [PMID: 22228948]

[105] Vasudevan P, Kashyap S, Sharma S. Bioactive botanicals from basil (*Ocimum* sp.). J Sci Indu Res 1999; 58: 332-8.

[106] Abou El-Soud NH, Deabes M, Abou El-Kassem L, Khalil M. Chemical Composition and Antifungal Activity of *Ocimum basilicum* L. Essential Oil. Open Access Maced J Med Sci 2015; 3(3): 374-9.
[http://dx.doi.org/10.3889/oamjms.2015.082] [PMID: 27275253]

[107] Kocić-Tanackova SD. Antifungal Activity of The Basil (Ocimmum Basilicum L.) Extract on Penicillium aurantiogriseum, P. glabrum, P. chrysogenum, and P. brevicompactum. Acta Period techn 2012; 43: 1-342.

[108] Khan A, Ahmad A, Manzoor N, Khan LA. Antifungal activities of *Ocimum sanctum* essential oil and its lead molecules. Nat Prod Commun 2010; 5(2): 1934578X1000500.
[http://dx.doi.org/10.1177/1934578X1000500235] [PMID: 20334156]

[109] Mondal S, Varma S, Bamola VD, *et al.* Double-blinded randomized controlled trial for immunomodulatory effects of Tulsi (*Ocimum sanctum* Linn.) leaf extract on healthy volunteers. J Ethnopharmacol 2011; 136(3): 452-6.
[http://dx.doi.org/10.1016/j.jep.2011.05.012] [PMID: 21619917]

[110] Shree P, Mishra P, Selvaraj C. Targeting COVID-19 (SARS-CoV-2) main protease through active phytochemicals of ayurvedic medicinal plants – Withania somnifera (Ashwagandha), Tinospora cordifolia (Giloy) and Ocimum sanctum (Tulsi) – A molecular docking study. J Biomol Struct Dyna 2020; 1-14.
[http://dx.doi.org/10.1080/07391102.2020.1810778]

[111] Kaya I, Yigit N, Benli M. Antimicrobial activity of various extracts of <i>Ocimum basilicum</i> l. and observation of the inhibition effect on bacterial cells by use of scanning electron microscopy. Afr J Tradit Complement Altern Med 2008; 5(4): 363-9.
[http://dx.doi.org/10.4314/ajtcam.v5i4.31291] [PMID: 20161958]

[112] Bonjar S. Evaluation of antibacterial properties of some medicinal plants used in Iran. J

Ethnopharmacol 2004; 94(2-3): 301-5.
[http://dx.doi.org/10.1016/j.jep.2004.06.007] [PMID: 15325735]

[113] Qureshi AA, Kumar KE. Phytochemical constituents and pharmacological activities of *Trachyspermum ammi*. Plant Arch 2010; 10: 955-9.

[114] Kaur GJ, Arora DS. *In vitro* antibacterial activity of three plants belonging to the family Umbelliferae. Int J Antimicrob Agents 2008; 31(4): 393-5.
[http://dx.doi.org/10.1016/j.ijantimicag.2007.11.007] [PMID: 18191549]

[115] Zaidi SFH, Yamada K, Kadowaki M, Usmanghani K, Sugiyama T. Bactericidal activity of medicinal plants, employed for the treatment of gastrointestinal ailments, against *Helicobacter pylori*. J Ethnopharmacol 2009; 121(2): 286-91.
[http://dx.doi.org/10.1016/j.jep.2008.11.001] [PMID: 19041711]

[116] Bonjar S. Evaluation of antibacterial properties of some medicinal plants used in Iran. J Ethnopharmacol 2004; 94(2-3): 301-5.
[http://dx.doi.org/10.1016/j.jep.2004.06.007] [PMID: 15325735]

[117] Khan NT, Jameel N. Antifungal Activity of Ajawain Seeds (Trachyspermum ammi). J Biomol Res Ther 2018; 7(2): 164.
[http://dx.doi.org/10.4172/2167-7956.1000164]

[118] Tripathi SC, Singh SP, Dube S. Studies on antifungal properties of essential oil of *Trachyspermum ammi* (L.) Sprague. J Phytopathol 1986; 116(2): 113-20.
[http://dx.doi.org/10.1111/j.1439-0434.1986.tb00902.x]

[119] Roy S, Chaurvedi P, Chowdhary A. Evaluation of antiviral activity of essential oil of *Trachyspermum Ammi* against Japanese encephalitis virus. Pharmacognosy Res 2015; 7(3): 263-7.
[http://dx.doi.org/10.4103/0974-8490.157977] [PMID: 26130938]

[120] Caccioni DRL, Guizzardi M, Biondi DM, Agatino Renda , Ruberto G. Relationship between volatile components of citrus fruit essential oils and antimicrobial action on *Penicillium digitatum* and *Penicillium italicum*. Int J Food Microbiol 1998; 43(1-2): 73-9.
[http://dx.doi.org/10.1016/S0168-1605(98)00099-3] [PMID: 9761340]

[121] Murthy PS, Borse BB, Khanum H, Srinivas P. Inhibitory effects of Ajwain (*Trachyspermum ammi*) ethanolic extract on *A. ochraceus* growth and ochratoxin production. Turk J Biol 2009; 33: 211-7. Corpus ID: 54512592.

[122] Yadav UCS, Baquer NZ. Pharmacological effects of *Trigonella foenum-graecum* L. in health and disease. Pharm Biol 2014; 52(2): 243-54.
[http://dx.doi.org/10.3109/13880209.2013.826247] [PMID: 24102093]

[123] Nasroallah MK, Kolsum M. Physiological and Pharmaceutical Effects of Fenugreek (*Trigonella foenum-graecum* L.) as a Multipurpose and Valuable Medicinal Plant. Glob J Med Plant Res 2013; 1(2): 199-206. Corpus ID: 7428969.

[124] Nandagopal S, Dhanalakshmi DP, Kumar AG, Sujitha D. Phytochemical and antibacterial studies of fenugreek *Trigonella foenum-graecum* L.-A multipurpose medicinal plant. J Pharm Res 2012; 5: 413-5. Corpus ID: 212558486.

[125] Sowmya P, Rajyalakshmi P. Hypocholesterolemic effect of germinated fenugreek seeds in human subjects. Plants foods Hum Nutr 1999; 53: 359-65.
[http://dx.doi.org/10.1023/a:1008021618733]

[126] Haouala R, Hawala S, El-Ayeb A, Khanfir R, Boughanmi N. Aqueous and organic extracts of *Trigonella foenum-graecum* L. inhibit the mycelia growth of fungi. J Environ Sci (China) 2008; 20(12): 1453-7.
[http://dx.doi.org/10.1016/S1001-0742(08)62548-6] [PMID: 19209631]

[127] Randhir R, Shetty K. Improved alpha-amylase and *Helicobacter pylori* inhibition by fenugreek extracts derived *via* solid-state bioconversion using *Rhizopus oligosporus*. Asia Pac J Clin Nutr 2007;

16(3): 382-92.
[PMID: 17704018]

[128] Dharmashekara C, Pradeep S, Prasad SK, *et al.* Virtual screening of potential phyto-candidates as therapeutic leads against SARS-CoV-2 infection. Environmental Challenges 2021; 4: 100136. [http://dx.doi.org/10.1016/j.envc.2021.100136]

[129] Byler KG, Ogungbe IV, Setzer WN. *In-silico* screening for anti-Zika virus phytochemicals. J Mol Graph Model 2016; 69: 78-91. [http://dx.doi.org/10.1016/j.jmgm.2016.08.011] [PMID: 27588363]

[130] Al-Asadi JN. Therapeutic uses of fenugreek (*Trigonella foenum-graecum* L.). Am J Soc Iss Hum 2014; 2: 21-36.

[131] Arokiyaraj S, Dinesh Kumar V, Elakya V, *et al.* Biosynthesized silver nanoparticles using floral extract of *Chrysanthemum indicum* L.—potential for malaria vector control. Environ Sci Pollut Res Int 2015; 22(13): 9759-65. [http://dx.doi.org/10.1007/s11356-015-4148-9] [PMID: 25637241]

[132] Lee JH, Van ND, Ma JY, Kim Y-B, Kim S-K, Paik H-D. Screening of antiviral medicinal plants against avian influenza virus H1N1 for food safety. Han-gug Chugsan Sigpum Hag-hoeji 2010; 30(2): 345-50. [http://dx.doi.org/10.5851/kosfa.2010.30.2.345]

[133] Hussein EA, Taj-Eldeen AM, Al-Zubairi AS, Elhakimi AS, Al-Dubaie AR. Phytochemical screening, Total phenolics and antioxidant and antibacterial activities of callus from *Brassica nigra* L. hypocotyl explants. Int J Pharmacol 2010; 6(4): 464-71. [http://dx.doi.org/10.3923/ijp.2010.464.471]

[134] Engels C, Schieber A, Gänzle MG. Sinapic acid derivatives in defatted Oriental mustard (Brassica juncea L.) seed meal extracts using UHPLC-DAD-ESI-MS n and identification of compounds with antibacterial activity. Eur Food Res Technol 2012; 234(3): 535-42. [http://dx.doi.org/10.1007/s00217-012-1669-z]

[135] Ogidi OI, George DG, Enenebeaku UE, Esie NG, Akpan UM. Efficacy evaluation of extracts of *Brassica juncea* (Brown mustard) seeds as potential antimicrobial agent against pathogenic microbes. J Med Plants Stud 2019; 7(4): 263-5. Corpus ID: 251312708.

[136] Clemente I, Aznar M, Silva F, Nerín C. Antimicrobial properties and mode of action of mustard and cinnamon essential oils and their combination against foodborne bacteria. Innov Food Sci Emerg Technol 2016; 36: 26-33. [http://dx.doi.org/10.1016/j.ifset.2016.05.013]

[137] Zhang Y. Cancer-preventive isothiocyanates: measurement of human exposure and mechanism of action. Mutat Res 2004; 555(1-2): 173-90. [http://dx.doi.org/10.1016/j.mrfmmm.2004.04.017] [PMID: 15476859]

[138] Dufour V, Stahl M, Baysse C. The antibacterial properties of isothiocyanates. Microbiology 2015; 161(2): 229-43. [http://dx.doi.org/10.1099/mic.0.082362-0] [PMID: 25378563]

[139] Borhade P, Lone K, Joshi S, Kadam A, Gaikwad P. Recent Pharmacological review of *Cinnamomum tamala.* Res J Pharm Biol Chem Sci 2013; 4(4): 916.

[140] Shah M, Panchal M. Ethanopharmacological Properties of *Cinnamomum tamala* – A Review. Int J Pharm Sci Rev Res 2010; 5(3): 141-4.

[141] Kumar S, Sharma S, Vasudeva N. Chemical compositions of *Cinnamomum tamala* oil from two different regions of India. Asian Pac J Trop Dis 2012; 2: S761-4. [http://dx.doi.org/10.1016/S2222-1808(12)60260-6]

[142] Parekh J, Chanda S. *In vitro* screening of antibacterial activity of aqueous and alcoholic extracts of various Indian plant species against selected pathogens from Enterobacteriaceae. Afr J Microbiol Res

2007; 1(6): 92-9. Corpus ID: 85718864

[143] Kapoor IPS, Singh B, Singh G, Isidorov VA, Szczepaniak L. Chemistry, antimicrobial and antioxidant potentials of *Cinnamomum tamala* Nees & Eberm. (Tejpat) essential oil and oleoresins. Nat Prod Radiance 2009; 8(2): 106-16. Corpus ID: 55373523.

[144] Sikkema J, de Bont JA, Poolman B. Interactions of cyclic hydrocarbons with biological membranes. J Biol Chem 1994; 269(11): 8022-8. [http://dx.doi.org/10.1016/S0021-9258(17)37154-5] [PMID: 8132524]

[145] Mishra AK, Singh BK, Pandey AK. *In vitro*-antibacterial activity and phytochemical profiles of *Cinnamomum tamala* (Tejpat) leaf extracts and oil. Rev Infect 2010; 1(3): 134-9.

[146] Farisa Banu S, Rubin D, Rakshitaa S, *et al.* Antivirulent properties of underexplored cinnamomum tamala essential oil and its synergistic effects with dnase against pseudomonas aeruginosa biofilms. An *In Vitro* Study. Front micro 2017; 8: 1144. [http://dx.doi.org/10.3389/fmicb.2017.01144]

[147] El-Ghorab AH, Javed Q, Anjum FM, Hamed SF, Shaaban HA. Pakistani bell pepper (*Capsicum annum* L.): Chemical compositions and its antioxidant activi-ty. Int J Food Prop 2013; 16(1): 18-32. [http://dx.doi.org/10.1080/10942912.2010.513616]

[148] Wahyuni Y, Ballester AR, Sudarmonowati E, Bino RJ, Bovy AG. Secondary metabolites of Capsicum species and their importance in the human diet. J Nat Prod 2013; 76(4): 783-93. [http://dx.doi.org/10.1021/np300898z] [PMID: 23477482]

[149] Soumya SL, Nair BR. Antifungal efficacy of *Capsicum frutescens* L. extracts against some prevalent fungal strains associated with groundnut storage. J Agric Technol 2012; 8(2): 739-50. Corpus ID: 26348554.

[150] Caterina MJ, Leffler A, Malmberg AB, *et al.* Impaired nociception and pain sensation in mice lacking the capsaicin receptor. Science 2000; 288(5464): 306-13. [http://dx.doi.org/10.1126/science.288.5464.306] [PMID: 10764638]

[151] Prasch S, Duran AG, Chinchilla N, Molinillo JMG, Macías FA, Bucar F. Resistance modulatory and efflux-inhibitory activities of capsaicinoids and capsinoids. Bioorg Chem 2019; 82: 378-84. [http://dx.doi.org/10.1016/j.bioorg.2018.10.062] [PMID: 30428416]

[152] Hafiz TA, Mubaraki MA, Dkhil MA, Al-Quraishy S. Antiviral Activities of *Capsicum annuum* Methanolic Extract against *Herpes Simplex* Virus 1 and 2. Pak J Zool 2017; 49(1): 251-5. [http://dx.doi.org/10.17582/journal.pjz/2017.49.1.251.255]

[153] Obi RK, Iroagba II, Ojiako OA. Virucidal potential of some edible Nigerian vegetables. Afr J Biotechnol 2006; 5: 1785-8. [http://dx.doi.org/10.4314/AJB.V5I19.55854]

[154] De Lucca AJ, Boue S, Palmgren MS, Maskos K, Cleveland TE. Fungicidal properties of two saponins from *Capsicum frutescens* and the relationship of structure and fungicidal activity. Can J Microbiol 2006; 52(4): 336-42. [http://dx.doi.org/10.1139/w05-137] [PMID: 16699584]

[155] Meriga B, Mopuri R, MuraliKrishna T. Insecticidal, antimicrobial and antioxidant activities of bulb extracts of Allium sativum. Asian Pac J Trop Med 2012; 5(5): 391-5. [http://dx.doi.org/10.1016/S1995-7645(12)60065-0] [PMID: 22546657]

[156] Wang HX, Ng TB. Purification of allivin, a novel antifungal protein from bulbs of the round-cloved garlic. Life Sci 2001; 70(3): 357-65. [http://dx.doi.org/10.1016/S0024-3205(01)01399-6] [PMID: 12005268]

[157] Appel E, Vallon-Eberhard A, Rabinkov A, *et al.* Therapy of murine pulmonary aspergillosis with antibody-alliinase conjugates and alliin. Antimicrob Agents Chemother 2010; 54(2): 898-906. [http://dx.doi.org/10.1128/AAC.01267-09] [PMID: 19949059]

[158] Ankri S, Mirelman D. Antimicrobial properties of allicin from garlic. Microbes Infect 1999; 1(2): 125-9.
[http://dx.doi.org/10.1016/S1286-4579(99)80003-3] [PMID: 10594976]

[159] Ogita A, Fujita K, Taniguchi M, Tanaka T. Enhancement of the fungicidal activity of amphotericin B by allicin, an allyl-sulfur compound from garlic, against the yeast *Saccharomyces cerevisiae* as a model system. Planta Med 2006; 72(13): 1247-50.
[http://dx.doi.org/10.1055/s-2006-947203] [PMID: 16902870]

[160] An M, Shen H, Cao Y, *et al.* Allicin enhances the oxidative damage effect of amphotericin B against *Candida albicans.* Int J Antimicrob Agents 2009; 33(3): 258-63.
[http://dx.doi.org/10.1016/j.ijantimicag.2008.09.014] [PMID: 19095412]

[161] Weber N, Andersen D, North J, Murray B, Lawson L, Hughes B. *In vitro* virucidal effects of *Allium sativum* (garlic) extract and compounds. Planta Med 1992; 58(5): 417-23.
[http://dx.doi.org/10.1055/s-2006-961504] [PMID: 1470664]

[162] Adetumbi M, Javor GT, Lau BH. *Allium sativum* (garlic) inhibits lipid synthesis by *Candida albicans.* Antimicrob Agents Chemother 1986; 30(3): 499-501.
[http://dx.doi.org/10.1128/AAC.30.3.499] [PMID: 3535667]

[163] Yoshida S, Kasuga S, Hayashi N, Ushiroguchi T, Matsuura H, Nakagawa S. Antifungal activity of ajoene derived from garlic. Appl Environ Microbiol 1987; 53(3): 615-7.
[http://dx.doi.org/10.1128/aem.53.3.615-617.1987] [PMID: 3555334]

[164] Rouf R, Uddin SJ, Sarker DK, *et al.* Antiviral potential of garlic (*Allium sativum*) and its organosulfur compounds: A systematic update of pre-clinical and clinical data. Trends Food Sci Technol 2020; 104: 219-34.
[http://dx.doi.org/10.1016/j.tifs.2020.08.006] [PMID: 32836826]

[165] Kshirsagar M, Dodamani A, Karibasappa G, *et al.* Antibacterial activity of garlic extract on cariogenic bacteria: An *in vitro* study. Ayu 2018; 39(3): 165-8.
[http://dx.doi.org/10.4103/ayu.AYU_193_16] [PMID: 31000994]

[166] Demin G, Yingying Z. Comparative antibacterial activities of crude polysaccharides and flavonoids from *Zingiber officinale* and their extraction. Am J Trop Med 2010; 5: 235-8. Corpus ID: 220862597.

[167] Grzanna R, Lindmark L, Frondoza CG. Ginger--an herbal medicinal product with broad anti-inflammatory actions. J Med Food 2005; 8(2): 125-32.
[http://dx.doi.org/10.1089/jmf.2005.8.125] [PMID: 16117603]

[168] Shukla Y, Singh M. Cancer preventive properties of ginger: A brief review. Food Chem Toxicol 2007; 45(5): 683-90.
[http://dx.doi.org/10.1016/j.fct.2006.11.002] [PMID: 17175086]

[169] Ali BH, Blunden G, Tanira MO, Nemmar A. Some phytochemical, pharmacological and toxicological properties of ginger (*Zingiber officinale* Roscoe): A review of recent research. Food Chem Toxicol 2008; 46(2): 409-20.
[http://dx.doi.org/10.1016/j.fct.2007.09.085] [PMID: 17950516]

[170] Govindarajan VS. Ginger--chemistry, technology, and quality evaluation: part 1. Crit Rev Food Sci Nutr 1982; 17(1): 1-96.
[PMID: 7049579]

[171] Zadeh JB, Kor NM. Physiological and pharmaceutical effects of Ginger (*Zingiber officinale* Roscoe) as a valuable medicinal plant. Eur J Exp Biol 2014; 4(1): 87-90. Corpus ID: 44221439

[172] Chang JS, Wang KC, Yeh CF, Shieh DE, Chiang LC. Fresh ginger (*Zingiber officinale*) has anti-viral activity against human respiratory syncytial virus in human respiratory tract cell lines. J Ethnopharmacol 2013; 145(1): 146-51.
[http://dx.doi.org/10.1016/j.jep.2012.10.043] [PMID: 23123794]

[173] Aldwihi LA, Khan SI, Alamri FF, *et al.* Patients' behaviour regarding dietary or herbal supplements before and during COVID-19 in Saudi Arabia. Int J Environ Res Public Health 2021; 18(10): 5086. [http://dx.doi.org/10.3390/ijerph18105086] [PMID: 34064950]

[174] El-Baroty GS, El-Baky HHA, Farag RS, Saleh MA. Characterization of antioxidant and antimicrobial compounds of cinnamon and ginger essential oils. Afr J Biochem Res 2010; 6: 167-74. Corpus ID: 53637648.

[175] Chandarana H, Baluja S, Chanda SV. Comparison of antibacterial activities of selected species of zingiberaceae family and some synthetic compounds. Turk J Biol 2005; 29: 83-97.

[176] Wang H, Ng TB. An antifungal protein from ginger rhizomes. Biochem Biophys Res Commun 2005; 336(1): 100-4. [http://dx.doi.org/10.1016/j.bbrc.2005.08.058] [PMID: 16125680]

[177] Abdel-Moneim A, Morsy BM, Mahmoud AM, Abo-Seif MA, Zanaty MI. Beneficial therapeutic effects of *Nigella sativa* and/or *Zingiber officinale* in HCV patients in Egypt. EXCLI J 2013; 12: 943-55. [PMID: 27298610]

[178] Oso BJ, Adeoye AO, Olaoye IF. Pharmacoinformatics and hypothetical studies on allicin, curcumin, and gingerol as potential candidates against COVID-19-associated proteases. J Biomol Struct Dyn 2022; 40(1): 389-400. [http://dx.doi.org/10.1080/07391102.2020.1813630] [PMID: 32876538]

[179] Ajay S, Rahul S, Sujit G, Paras M, Mishra A, Gaurav A. Comprehensive review: *Murraya koenigii* Linn. Asian J Pharm Life Sci 2007; 1(4): 417-25. Corpus ID: 74688265.

[180] Balunas MJ, Kinghorn AD. Drug discovery from medicinal plants. Life Sci 2005; 78(5): 431-41. [http://dx.doi.org/10.1016/j.lfs.2005.09.012] [PMID: 16198377]

[181] Ramadas D, Kowti R, Ramesh B, Nune SV, Joshi S. Antibacterial protection of polyphenols from curry leaves (Murraya koenigii): A research study. Int J Innov Sci Technol 2020; 5(10): 1281-3.

[182] Naik SK, Mohanty S, Padhi A, Pati R, Sonawane A. Evaluation of antibacterial and cytotoxic activity of *Artemisia nilagirica* and *Murraya koenigii* leaf extracts against mycobacteria and macrophages. BMC Complement Altern Med 2014; 14(1): 87. [http://dx.doi.org/10.1186/1472-6882-14-87] [PMID: 24597853]

[183] Disegha GC, Onuegbu IV. Antifungal Activities of Curry Leaf (*Murraya koengii*) Extract on Some Selected Fungi. Chem Mater Res 2014; 6(11): 2224-3224. Corpus ID: 54620086.

[184] Alalwan H, Rajendran R, Lappin DF, *et al.* The anti-adhesive effect of curcumin on *Candida albicans* biofilms on denture materials. Front Microbiol 2017; 8: 659. [http://dx.doi.org/10.3389/fmicb.2017.00659] [PMID: 28473808]

[185] Bhandari P. Curry leaf (*Murraya koenigii*) or Cure leaf: Review of its curative properties. Journal of Medical Nutrition and Nutraceuticals 2012; 1(2): 92-7. [http://dx.doi.org/10.4103/2278-019X.101295]

[186] El-Amin M, Virk P, Elobeid MAR, *et al.* Anti-diabetic effect of Murraya koenigii (L) and Olea europaea (L) leaf extracts on streptozotocin induced diabetic rats. Pak J Pharm Sci 2013; 26(2): 359-65. [PMID: 23455208]

[187] Kregiel D, Berłowska J, Witońska IA. Saponine-based, biological-active surfactants from plants. In: Najjar E, Ed. Application and characterization of surfactants. InTech 2017; pp. 183-205. [http://dx.doi.org/10.5772/68062]

[188] Wang GW, Hu WT, Huang BK, Qin LP. *Illicium verum*: A review on its botany, traditional use, chemistry and pharmacology. J Ethnopharmacol 2011; 136(1): 10-20. [http://dx.doi.org/10.1016/j.jep.2011.04.051] [PMID: 21549817]

[189] Hirschfeld G, Weber L, Renkl A, Scharffetter-Kochanek K, Weiss JM. Anaphylaxis after Oseltamivir (Tamiflu ®) therapy in a patient with sensitization to star anise and celery-carrot-mugwort-spice syndrome. Allergy 2008; 63(2): 243-4.
[http://dx.doi.org/10.1111/j.1398-9995.2007.01572.x] [PMID: 18186817]

[190] Hanif MA, Nisar S, Akhtar MN, Nisar N, Rashid N. Optimized production and advanced assessment of biodiesel: A review. Int J Energy Res 2018; 42(6): 2070-83.
[http://dx.doi.org/10.1002/er.3990]

[191] Yan J, Xiao X, Huang K. Component analysis of volatile oil from *Illicium Verum* Hook. f. J Cent South Univ Technol 2002; 9(3): 173-6.
[http://dx.doi.org/10.1007/s11771-002-0021-3]

[192] Aly SE, Sabry BA, Shaheen MS, Hathout AS. Assessment of antimycotoxigenic and antioxidant activity of star anise. J Saudi Soci Agri Sci 2016; 15(1): 20-7.
[http://dx.doi.org/10.1016/J.JSSAS.2014.05.003]

[193] Song WY, Ma YB, Bai X, *et al.* Two new compounds and anti-HIV active constituents from *Illicium verum.* Planta Med 2007; 73(4): 372-5.
[http://dx.doi.org/10.1055/s-2007-967162] [PMID: 17394104]

[194] Brochot A, Guilbot A, Haddioui L, Roques C. Antibacterial, antifungal, and antiviral effects of three essential oil blends. MicrobiologyOpen 2017; 6(4): e00459.
[http://dx.doi.org/10.1002/mbo3.459] [PMID: 28296357]

[195] Koch C, Reichling J, Schneele J, Schnitzler P. Inhibitory effect of essential oils against *herpes simplex* virus type 2. Phytomedicine 2008; 15(1-2): 71-8.
[http://dx.doi.org/10.1016/j.phymed.2007.09.003] [PMID: 17976968]

[196] Abdallah MH, Sobhy H, Enan G. Evaluation of antiviral activity of selected anise oil as an essential oil against bovine herpes virus type -1 *in vitro.* Glob Vet 2013; 10(5): 496-9.

[197] Alhajj MS, Qasem MA, Al-Mufarrej SI. Inhibitory Activity of *Illicium verum* Extracts against Avian Viruses. Adv Virol 2020; 2020: 1-8.
[http://dx.doi.org/10.1155/2020/4594635] [PMID: 32411246]

[198] Marcucci MC, Ferreres F, García-Viguera C, *et al.* Phenolic compounds from Brazilian propolis with pharmacological activities. J Ethnopharmacol 2001; 74(2): 105-12.
[http://dx.doi.org/10.1016/S0378-8741(00)00326-3] [PMID: 11167028]

[199] Conner DE, Davidson PT, Branen AL. Naturally occurring compounds. Antimicrobials in foods. New York: Marcel Dekker 1993; p. 54.

[200] Kim J, Marshall MR, Wei C. Antibacterial activity of some essential oil components against five foodborne pathogens. J Agric Food Chem 1995; 43(11): 2839-45.
[http://dx.doi.org/10.1021/jf00059a013]

[201] Alhajj MS, Qasem MAA, Nabi ARJE, Al-Mufarrej SI. *In-Vitro* Antibacterial and Antifungal Effects of High Levels of Chinese Star Anise. Brazilian Journal of Poultry Science 2019; 21(1): eRBCA-2019-0427.
[http://dx.doi.org/10.1590/1806-9061-2016-0427]

[202] Huang Y, Zhao J, Zhou L, *et al.* Antifungal activity of the essential oil of *Illicium verum* fruit and its main component trans-anethole. Molecules 2010; 15(11): 7558-69.
[http://dx.doi.org/10.3390/molecules15117558] [PMID: 21030909]

[203] Chattopadhyay I, Biswas K, Bandyopadhyay U, Banerjee RK. Turmeric and curcumin: Biological actions and medicinal applications. Curr Sci 2004; 87: 44-50.

[204] Abas F, Lajis NH, Shaari K, *et al.* A labdane diterpene glucoside from the rhizomes of Curcuma mangga. J Nat Prod 2005; 68(7): 1090-3.
[http://dx.doi.org/10.1021/np0500171] [PMID: 16038556]

[205] Syu WJ, Shen CC, Don MJ, Ou JC, Lee GH, Sun CM. Cytotoxicity of curcuminoids and some novel compounds from *Curcuma zedoaria*. J Nat Prod 1998; 61(12): 1531-4. [http://dx.doi.org/10.1021/np980269k] [PMID: 9868158]

[206] Mohamad H, Lajis NH, Abas F, *et al.* Antioxidative constituents of *Etlingera elatior*. J Nat Prod 2005; 68(2): 285-8. [http://dx.doi.org/10.1021/np040098l] [PMID: 15730265]

[207] Akram M, Shahab-Uddin Khan AA, Chani U, Hanan A, Mohiuddin E, Asif M. *Curcuma longa* and Curcumin- A review article. Rom J Biol Plant Biol 2010; 55: 65-72.

[208] Aggarwal BB, Sundram C, Malani N, Ichikawa H. Curcumin: The Indian Solid Gold. Curr Sci 2010; 332: 16-34. [http://dx.doi.org/10.1007/978-0-387-46401-5_1.]

[209] Araújo CAC, Leon LL. Biological activities of *Curcuma longa* L. Mem Inst Oswaldo Cruz 2001; 96(5): 723-8. [http://dx.doi.org/10.1590/S0074-02762001000500026] [PMID: 11500779]

[210] Gujral ML, Chowdhury NK, Saxena PN. The effect of certain indigenous remedies on the healing of wounds and ulcers. J Indian Med Assoc 1953; 22(7): 273-6. [PMID: 13052942]

[211] Niamsa N, Sittiwet C. Antimicrobial activity of *Curcuma longa* aqueous extract. J Pharmacol Toxicol 2009; 4(4): 173-7. [http://dx.doi.org/10.3923/jpt.2009.173.177]

[212] Ungphaiboon S, Supavita T, Singchangchai P, Sungkarak S, Rattanasuwan P, Itharat A. Study on antioxidant and antimicrobial activities of turmeric clear liquid soap for wound treatment of HIV patients. Songklanakarin J Sci Technol 2005; 27(2): 269-578. Corpus ID: 54635247.

[213] Lawhavinit OA, Kongkathip N, Kongkathip B. Antimicrobial activity of curcuminoids from Curcuma longa L. on pathogenic bacteria of shrimp and chicken. Witthayasan kasetsart 2010; 44(3): 346-71. Corpus ID: 3587077.

[214] Tajbakhsh S, Mohammadi K, Deilami I, *et al.* Antibacterial activity of indium curcumin and indium diacetylcurcumin. Afr J Biotechnol 2008; 7(21): 3832-5. [http://dx.doi.org/10.5897/AJB08.790]

[215] Moghadamtousi SZ, Kadir HA, Hassandarvish P, Tajik H, Abubakar S, Zandi K. A review on antibacterial, antiviral, and antifungal activity of curcumin. BioMed Res Int 2014; 2014: 186864. [PMID: 24877064]

[216] Tahmasebi S, El-Esawi MA, Mahmoud ZH, *et al.* Immunomodulatory effects of nanocurcumin on Th17 cell responses in mild and severe COVID-19 patients. J Cell Physiol 2021; 236(7): 5325-38. [http://dx.doi.org/10.1002/jcp.30233] [PMID: 33372280]

[217] Valizadeh H, Abdolmohammadi-vahid S, Danshina S, *et al.* Nano-curcumin therapy, a promising method in modulating inflammatory cytokines in COVID-19 patients. Int Immunopharmacol 2020; 89(Pt B): 107088. [http://dx.doi.org/10.1016/j.intimp.2020.107088] [PMID: 33129099]

[218] Adamczak A, Ożarowski M, Karpiński TM. Curcumin, a natural antimicrobial agent with strain-specific activity. Pharmaceuticals 2020; 13(7): 153. [http://dx.doi.org/10.3390/ph13070153] [PMID: 32708619]

[219] Tyagi P, Singh M, Kumari H, Kumari A, Mukhopadhyay K. Bactericidal activity of curcumin I is associated with damaging of bacterial membrane. PLoS One 2015; 10(3): e0121313. [http://dx.doi.org/10.1371/journal.pone.0121313] [PMID: 25811596]

CHAPTER 3

Role of Herbal Medicines in the Treatment of Infectious Diseases

Ramesh S. Chaughule[1,*] and **Rajesh S. Barve**[2]

[1] *Department of Chemistry, Ramnarain Ruia Autonomous College, Matunga, Mumbai 400019, India*

[2] *Department of Repertory, Virar Homeopathic Medical College, Virar East, Maharashtra, 401303, India*

Abstract: Herbal medicines have helped to cure illness because the practice has continued for generations. Multiple alkaloids/compounds that occur naturally (as against single extracts) exhibit synergistic action and do not show antidote action. This naturally occurring combination of compounds exhibits antiviral, antibacterial, antiprotozoal, and antioxidant actions. The cases related to viral, protozoal, and bacterial infections were selected. Patients with amoebiasis, *e-coli*, gastrointestinal infection, skin and urinary tract infections were treated using herbal drugs. Diagnoses were confirmed with investigations. Repeated investigations were carried out to confirm the improvement.

Most herbal medicines do not exhibit serious side effects and are safe to prescribe, showing greater acceptability. Thus, due to their cost effectiveness, these medicines are in great demand for primary health care for better cultural acceptability and minimal side effects.

Cases varying from COVID 19 to gastrointestinal infection, viral diseases, and skin and wound infections are being treated effectively with herbal drugs.

Keywords: Aegle Folia, Aspidosperma, Alkaloids, Bryonia alba, COVID 19, Eupatorium perfoliatum, Herbal medicines, Holarrhena Antidysenterica, Infectious diseases, *In vitro* studies, Justicia.

1. INTRODUCTION

The use of herbal medicines for the treatment of various health challenges continues to expand rapidly across the world with many people now resorting to these products for improved healthcare.

* **Corresponding author Ramesh S. Chaughule:** Department of Chemistry, Ramnarain Ruia Autonomous College, Matunga, Mumbai 400019, India; E-mail: rsctifr@yahoo.com

Atta-ur-Rahman & Ka Bian (Eds.)

There is a tremendous surge in acceptance and public interest in natural therapies both in developing and developed countries, with these herbal remedies being available not only in drug stores but also in food stores. Herbal medicinal products are the primary healthcare source for the large population living in developing countries. India has a rich traditional system of medicine. Therapeutic treatments like Ayurveda, Unani, Homeopathy, Sidha, *etc* use mostly herbs. Natural herbal products are being used for the development of modern drugs and dietary supplements to food and beverages. Thus, traditional medicines to have provided a good level of confidence in safety and efficacy as the medicines have been used for thousands of years. There is a growing interest in natural products as a source of new chemical entities for the development of modern drugs and the use of natural products as dietary supplements, ingredients for food and beverages, Phyto cosmetics, and other herbal products.

Herbal medicine is a botanical product that can be used in extract or dilution form. The usage increases when conventional medicine is ineffective because of the growing drug resistance. Large numbers of plant species are used by the Indian herbal industry. These medicines are the synthesis of the therapeutic experiences of generations of practicing physicians. Multiple alkaloids/compounds that occur naturally (as against single extracts) show synergistic action and do not show antidote action. The naturally occurring combinations of compounds exhibit antiviral, antibacterial, antiprotozoal, and antioxidant actions. The cases related to viral, protozoal, and bacterial infections were selected. Patients with amoebiasis, *e-coli*, gastrointestinal infection, skin and urinary tract infections were treated using herbal drugs. Diagnoses were confirmed with investigations. Repeated investigations were carried out to confirm the improvement. Drug and plant review of herbal medicines used is also described in the text.

Since people are more worried about using conventional medicines due to their growing drug resistance, they continue to use traditional herbal medicines for good healthcare. Many hundreds of plants worldwide are used in traditional medicine for the treatment of bacterial infections. Some of these have also been subjected to *in vitro* screening but the efficacy of such herbal medicines has seldom been rigorously tested in controlled clinical trials. Bacterial infection is another source of problem for mankind. Though conventional medicines have effective antibiotic therapy for bacterial infection, they have drug resistance problems. Hence, many known plants are used globally for the treatment of bacterial infections. Thus, healthcare practitioners must be aware of herbal antibiotics. The present study is undertaken to assess critically those antibacterial herbal medicines that have been subjected to controlled clinical trials.

1.1. Pharmacology

Pharmacology can be defined as the therapy of the interaction of biologically active agents with living systems [1] and is further divided into two main areas pharmacodynamics and pharmacokinetics. Pharmacodynamics looks at the effects of an agent at active sites in the body. In contrast, pharmacokinetics is concerned with the medicinal effect on the body. For the therapeutic study, the aim is to examine the pharmacology of key chemical groups in plants as individual herbs under phytochemistry. Nutrients such as vitamins, minerals, and so on are largely responsible for the pharmacological activity of plants.

1.2. Secondary Metabolites

Primary metabolites participate in nutrition and essential metabolic processes inside the plant, whereas secondary metabolites influence ecological interactions between the plant and its environment. Based on their biosynthetic origins, plant secondary metabolites can be divided into three major groups: terpenoids, alkaloids, phenylpropanoid, and allied phenolic compounds [2]. All terpenoids, including the primary metabolites, are derived from the five-carbon precursor isopentenyl diphosphate. Alkaloids are biosynthesized from amino acids and phenolic compounds by either the shikimic acid pathway or the malonate/acetate pathway [2]. Two large groups of secondary plant metabolites can be distinguished in terms of their biological/therapeutic activities, as suggested by Efferth and Koch [3].

1.3. Herbal Medicines and Conventional Drugs

Though conventional drugs or their precursors are derived from plants, there is a fundamental difference between administering a pure chemical and the same chemical in a plant matrix. The homeopathic practitioner uses drugs in complex formulations, whereas a conventional physician prescribes a single agent. It does seem logical that, just as our foods are chemically complex, so should be our medicines. There are, however, several phytotherapy examples from the literature of how an advantage might arise from chemical complexity, and some of these are discussed below.

Synergy is an effect seen by a combination of substances that is greater than would have been expected from a consideration of individual contributions [4]. It is an important hypothesis in herbal pharmacology in the context of the advantage of chemical complexity. If the action of a chemical mixture is greater than the arithmetical sum of the actions of the mixture's components, the entire action is greater than the sum of the individual parts which can be considered as a cooperative or facilitating effect between the components for a specific outcome

[4]. In other words; components of plants that are not active themselves can act to improve the stability, solubility, bioavailability, or half-life of the active components. Hence, a particular chemical in pure form may have only a fraction of the pharmacological activity that it has in its plant matrix. This key mechanism for synergy, therefore, has a pharmacokinetic basis.

2. INFECTIOUS DISEASES

2.1. Amoebiasis, Giardiasis (Gastrointestinal illness)

Diarrhea and dysentery are common gastrointestinal disorders in tropical countries and especially in Asian countries. They contribute enormously in terms of morbidity and mortality. Worldwide more than 1 billion people suffer from acute diarrhea. In developing countries, it amounts to over 2-3 million deaths per year. Amoebiasis has emerged as a major health problem worldwide. It is endemic in the present scenario and different in sub-tropical regions, especially in Asia. It is an infectious disease which originated with the single-celled parasitic protozoan *Entamoeba histolytica.* The parasitic amoeba infects the liver and intestine and may cause mild diarrhea and serious dysentery with bloody and mucoid stool. Giardiasis is a common illness caused by a parasite that may result in diarrhea and stomach cramps. It is an infection in the small intestine and caused by a microscopic parasite called *Giardia lamblia*. The Giardia parasite can spread through contaminated water, food, and surfaces and from contact with someone who has it. Common organisms causing acute diarrhea are *E. coli, shigella, vibrio cholera, staph, aureus, giardia, salmonella, protozoa* like *Entamoeba histolytica*, and viruses like Rotavirus. Their average incubation period is less than 3-4 days. Pain in the abdomen, vomiting, and fever are the main causes of diarrhea. Major complications arise from fluid and electrolyte imbalance due to loss of fluid and dehydration [5].

Herbal/homeopathic medicines discussed below have an excellent response to these conditions of diarrhea and dysentery and no other medicines are required to treat these acute diseases. The results on the patients are given in Table **1**. The medicines Holarrhena *Antidysenterica* and *Aegle folia* are given in tincture form, which is ethanolic (90%) and drug strength of 1/10 as advised by homeopathic pharmacopeia of India. The efficacy of some of them is also tested *in vitro* to validate the results [6, 7].

Table 1. Gastro-Intestinal Infections Treated with Herbal Tinctures.

S. No	Sex/ Age	Clinical Presentation	Investigations	Drug and Dose	Result
1	M/ 45	Diabetic, history of outside food 10-12 loose stools/day Pain, cramps, dysentery abdomen, flatulens++	Stool: mucus++, watery stools pus cells 10-15, RBC +, e. histolytica+ RBC 180,	*Aegle folia* tincture 10 drops 4 times	Diarrhea frequency reduced in 1 day no diarrhea after 24 hrs
2	F/ 68	History of stale tin food, vomiting, pain abdomen+ bloating+ The next day watery diarrhea 6-8 / day. nausea, acidity +	CBC: WBC 11000, n: 80, 1 12. stool: watery, offensive, RBC +, WBC 10-12	*Holarrhena antidysenterica* tincture. 15 drops 4 times	Watery stool better in 24 hrs, frequency reduced to 2-3/day no diarrhea after 36 hrs
3	M/8	Swimming in the pool. Pain abdomen, vomiting on day one, followed by unformed stools next day, 3-4 /day for 4 days	Stool: giardia ++, mucus ++, RBC +	*Aegle folia* tincture. 10 drops 3 times	The stool improved in 2 days. Stool examination after 5 days. No giardia seen
4	M/ 1yr	History of travel, outside water taken. watery stools 12-15/day, loud, offensive poor appetite, vomiting +, fever 100f, Anal redness, excoriation min. dehydration	Stools: watery, yellowish, offensive, pus cells 15-20 Epithelial cells: 6-8 RBC++ *E. coli*	*Aegle folia* tincture. 5 drops + Holarrhena tincture 5 drops with water 4 times	With medicine and ors stool frequency reduced in 24 hrs and no diarrhea after 2 days.
5	M/65	History of dm, recurrent UTI, dysuria, fever recurrent diarrhea, weight loss, uncontrolled sugar, HbA1C: 8.6	Stool culture: *E. coli* colony count100000 resistant to common antibiotics	*Aegle folia* tincture 8 drops + Holarrhena tincture 8 drops 4 times	Fever and diarrhea improved in 2 days and culture-negative in 6 days

2.1.1. Holarrhena Antidysenterica (H.A.) [Family name: Apocynaceae]

H.A. is commonly called Kutaja in India (Fig. **1**). The plant grows wild in the mountains, in the tropical Himalayas, going up to an altitude of 1200 m. Also, these are found throughout many forests of India, such as Travancore, Assam, and Uttar Pradesh. It is an herb of choice for Amoebic dysentery. Kutaja (root, stem, and leaf) removes the amoeba from the body, which can cause severe problems like liver abscess. It can also be used for a natural cure of chronic diarrhea and dysentery and maintains the normalcy of the digestive system. The presence of alkaloids, phenolics, tannins, and triterpenoid-related compounds are identified through preliminary phytochemical tests. Thus, this drug inhibits acetylcholinesterase conessine, iso conessine, holarrhine, kurchamide and holarrhifin [8].

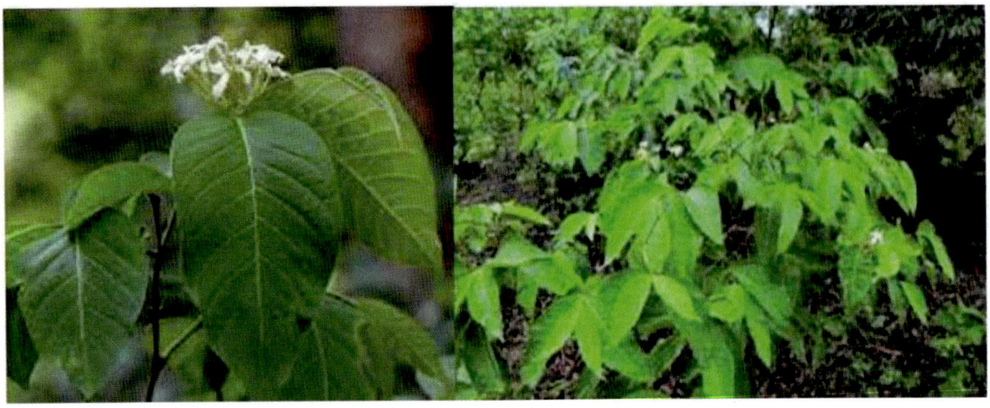

Fig. (1). Kutaja ***Aegle folia*** (wood apple or Bael) [Family name: *Rutaceae*].

These observations are authenticated through pharmacognostic studies by applying the specific stains on fresh freehand cross-sections of the stem tissue.

2.1.2. Aegle folia (Wood Apple or Bael) [Family name: Rutaceae]

It is a perennial woody tree grown in kitchen gardens, boundary plantations around mango orchards, and forest plantations in most of the states of India (Fig. **2**). *Aegle* belongs to one of the three monotypic genera of orange subfamily *Aurantioideae*, tribe *Clauseneae,* and subtribe *Balsamocitrinae*. *Aegle marmelos* Correa is deciduous, 6–8 meters in height with trifoliate aromatic leaves. The branches sometimes bear long straight spines. The bisexual flowers are nearly 2 cm wide, borne in clusters, sweet-scented, and greenish-white. Fruits are 5–7.5 cm in diameter, globose, oblong pyriform, rind gray or yellow, pulp sweet, and thick yellow, orange to brown in color. Seeds are numerous and arranged in the cells surrounded by slimy transparent mucilage.

Certain biochemical constituents, namely alkaloids, coumarin, and steroid are isolated from different parts of the Bael tree. These are Skimmianine, aegelin, Y-sitosterol, Aegelenine, Myrlene, p-menth-l-en-3 beta, 5 beta diol, N-2 phenyl ethyl cinnamate, N-hydroxy ethyl cinnamide, N-4 methoxystyryl cinnamate, N-2-hydroxy ethyl cinnamate, lupeol, sitosterol, Alloimperatorin, Imperatorin, ß-sitosterol, Marmesin, ß-sitosterol, Dietammine, Marmin, Umbelliferone, Lupeol, Marmelosin [9].

Inhibition of multiple sars cov2 protein by anti-viral molecule seselin occurs from *Aegle marmelos* and deciphers using molecular docking analysis. Seselin has the inhibitory potential over multiple sars cov2 targets and holds a high potential to work effectively as a novel drug for covid 19 [7, 9].

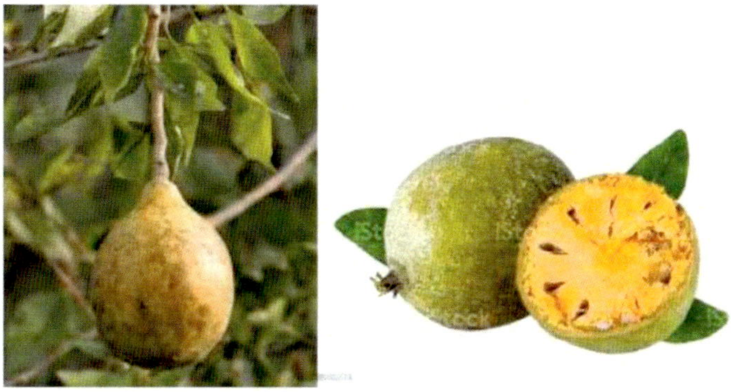

Fig. (2). Bael.

Clinical results carried out on patients who suffered from gastrointestinal infections are shown in Table **1**. Patients were treated with different herbal tinctures. Stool culture was taken from the patients having gastrointestinal infections. *S. aureus* was isolated as a causative organism. Sensitivity studies were done with a homeopathic herbal solution (0.1 ML) with a 5 mm sterile culture disc. 90% alcohol was kept as a standard as tinctures are hydro-alcoholic. Zone of inhibition was studied in comparison with alcohol disc. Disc with the combination of *Aegle Folia* and H.A. showed maximum zone of inhibition. This experiment is shown in Fig. (**3**). A similar *in vitro* experiment was performed using *E. coli* culture and depicted in Fig. (**4**).

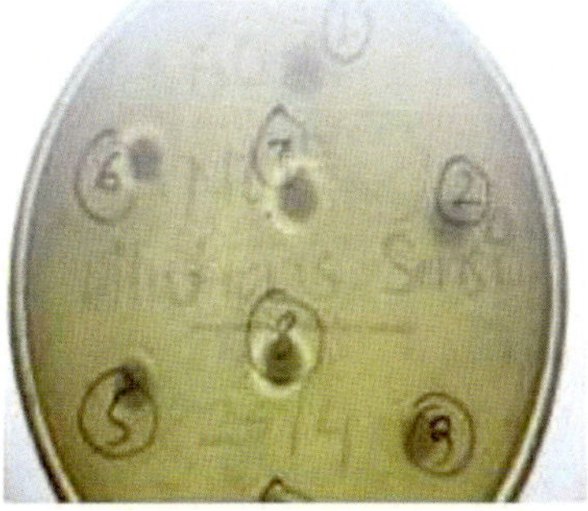

Fig. (3). *Staph. Aur.* Culture: **1**) Cynodon tincture, **2**) Echinesia tincture, **3**) Gambogia tincture, **4**) Podophyllum tincture, **5**) Ethanol control, **6**) *Aegle folia* tincture **7**) Holarrhena tincture **8**) *Aegle folia* + Holarrhena tincture.

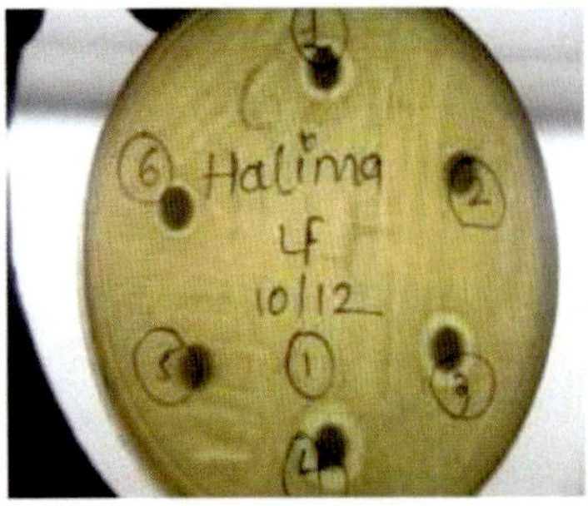

Fig. (4). **1**) *Aegle folia* tincture, **2**) Azardichata tincture, **3**) Holarrhena tincture, **4**) *Aegle folia* + Holarrhena tincture, **5**) Cynodon tincture, **6**) Ethanol control southeast corner.

2.2. Wound Healing

The wound is an anatomical and functional disruption of the skin following an injury. In response to the injury, wound healing is a complex process of tissue repair or remodeling. Wound care is constantly evolving with the advances in medicine. Platelets with fibrin help in clot formation at the injury site. Mediators of inflation are released along with the cellular response primarily at neutrophils and granular sites, which help in wound healing. Herbal medicines have been used by Ayurvedic practitioners and folk medicine practitioners for thousands of years.

In the current times, different types of biopolymers are being researched for developing economical, sustainable, stable, and effective delivery systems for the treatment of wounds. Recent scientific evidence and clinical trials conducted using traditional and alternative medicine in wound therapy hold good promise in the future.

2.2.1. Calendula

Calendula (*Calendula officinalis*) is a plant known as pot marigold [10]. It is a genus of about 15–20 species of annual and perennial herbaceous plants in the daisy family *Asteraceae* that are often known as marigolds [11]. They are native to southwestern Asia, Western Europe, Macaronesia, and the Mediterranean. The flowers of *C. officinalis* contain flavonol glycosides, triterpene oligoglycosides, oleanane type triterpene glycosides, saponins, and a sesquiterpene glucoside [12, 13].

Calendula officinalis oil is still used medicinally as an anti-inflammatory and a remedy for healing wounds in homeopathic and herbal literature [14]. Calendula ointments are skin products available for use on minor cuts, burns, and skin irritation [15].

Plant pharmacological studies have suggested that Calendula extracts have antiviral, antigenotoxic, and anti-inflammatory properties *in vitro* [16]. In herbalism, Calendula in suspension or in tincture is used topically for treating acne, reducing inflammation, controlling bleeding, and soothing irritated tissue. Topical application of *C. officinalis* ointment has helped prevent dermatitis and pain [17]. Calendula is being used traditionally for abdominal cramps and constipation. Calendula ethanolic tincture is used locally as an anti-inflammatory and step tic agent. The aqueous-ethanol extract of *C. officinalis* flowers shows both spasmolytic and spasmogenic effects, thus providing a scientific rationale for this traditional use [18].

2.2.2. Echinacea

Echinacea, also known as the purple coneflower, is an herbal medicine that has been used for centuries, customarily as a treatment for the common cold, coughs, bronchitis, upper respiratory infections [19], and some inflammatory conditions. Echinacea is promoted as a dietary supplement for the common cold and other infections, based on the idea that it might stimulate the immune system to more effectively fight infection. Echinacea preparations have been promoted for topical use (application to the skin) for wounds and skin problems. Current evidence indicates that the risk of interactions between echinacea supplements and most medications is low.

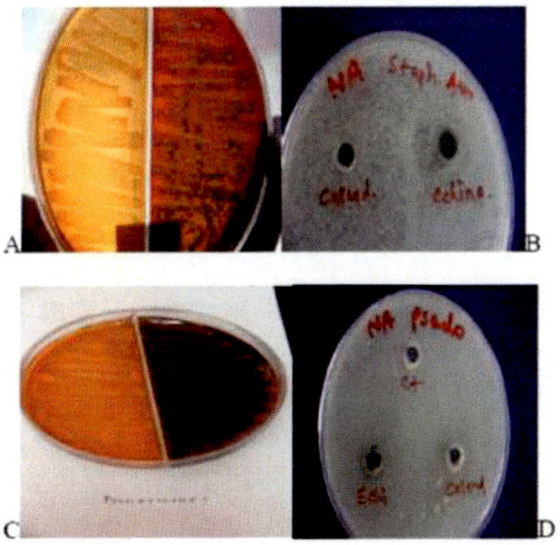

Fig. (5). *Pseudomonas* and *staph. aureus* are common pyogenic bacterias associated with wound infections which can cause delayed healing. Calendula and Echinacea effectively treat these infections and help wound healing. **(A)** *Staph. aureus* culture plate **(B)** *Staph. aureus*. sensitivity for Calendula and Echinacea **(C)** *Pseudomonas* culture **(D)** *Pseudomonas* sensitivity to Calendula and Echinacea.

The antibacterial activity of marigold (*calendula officinalis*) extract and echinacea on two reference strains, namely *staphylococcus aureus*, and *pseudomonas aeruginosa* were investigated (Fig. **5**). From the present study, it is seen that there is the most antibacterial activity of marigold methanolic extract and essential oil on gram-positive bacteria. For *Pseudomonas* and *staph. aureus,* the most active medicine is tincture (1:10) with 90% alcohol for the exhibition of highest activity. *Pseudomonas* and *staph. aureus* is common pyogenic bacteria associated with wound infections, which can cause delayed healing. Calendula and echinacea effectively treat these infections and help wound healing.

2.3. Epidemics

2.3.1. Dengue

Dengue is a mosquito-borne viral infection. Dengue virus is transmitted by female mosquitoes mainly of the species *Aedes aegypti* and, to a lesser extent, *Aedes albopictus*. The mosquitoes are vectors of chikungunya, yellow fever and Zika viruses. It is found in tropical and sub-tropical climates worldwide, mostly in urban and semi-urban areas. About half of the world's population is now at risk. The global incidence of dengue has grown dramatically in recent decades. Dengue is prevalent in Asian and African countries where the climate is humid and there is poor sanitation. The patient generally suffers from severe headache, pain behind the eyes, muscle and joint pains, nausea, vomiting, rash, *etc.*

Dengue is a viral fever. Viruses such as Arbo virus, RNA virus are transmitted by *Aedes aegypti* mosquito, in tropical countries, typically in monsoon season. After incubation period of 2-7 days, patient gets symptoms of fever, headache, body and muscle pains and retro orbital pains called as break-bone fever. A macular rash appears after 3-4 days. Illness typically lasts for 7-8 days. The illness can cause complications like thrombocytopenia, epistaxis, dengue hemorrhagic, and dengue shock syndrome. The fatality rate can be up to 8% [20].

Following are a few dengue cases treated effectively at the clinic in Mumbai in the dengue epidemic of 2014. The commonest herbal medicines used were (1) *Eupatorium Perfoliatum* and (2) *Bryonia alba.*

***Eupatorium Perfoliatum* Tincture** [Family: *Asteraceae*]. The tree (Fig. **6**) commonly called snakeroot or boneset, is a genus of flowering plants in the aster family, containing about 30 to 60 species depending on the classification system. The perennial plant is native to US and Canada, growing to almost 4 meters. Stem and flowers contain plant chemicals such as Eupafolin, curcumin, Rutin, Kaempferol, Quercetin, Gurgunen and are generally used for dengue, viral fever, and flu [21 - 24].

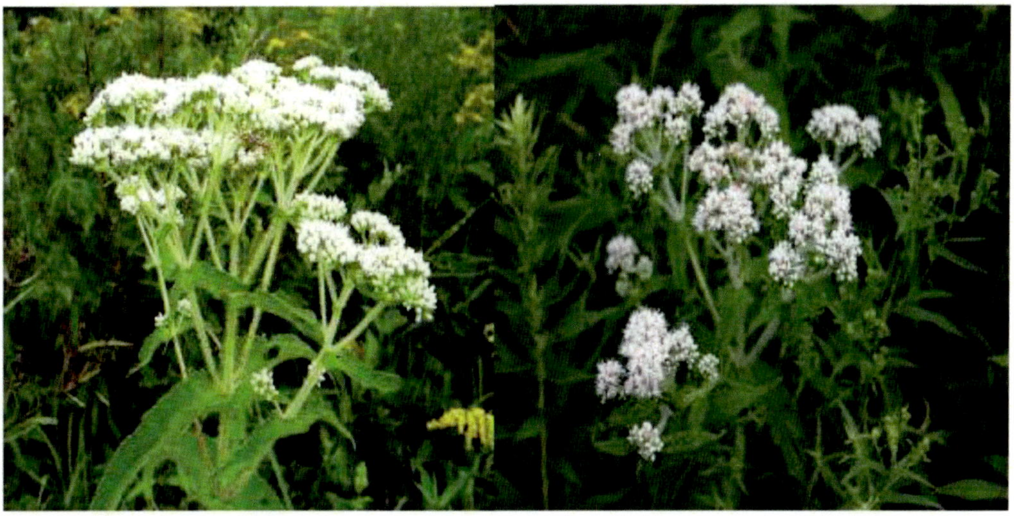

Fig. (6). *Eupatorium Perfoliatum.*

Bryonia tincture [Family: *B. alba*]. Bryonia is a plant in the gourd family (Fig. **7**). This perennial climbing vine has white flowers, red berries, and a thick, fleshy root with a strong, bitter odor. Its root is used as a medicine to prevent infection and to treat several diseases like intestinal diseases, lung diseases, arthritis, liver disease, and metabolic disorders; the appropriate dose of bryonia depends on several factors such as patient's age, health, and several other conditions. As a Homeopathic medicine, it is used for the treatment of dengue and relieves muscle and joint pain in the body with no side effects and no known drug interactions.

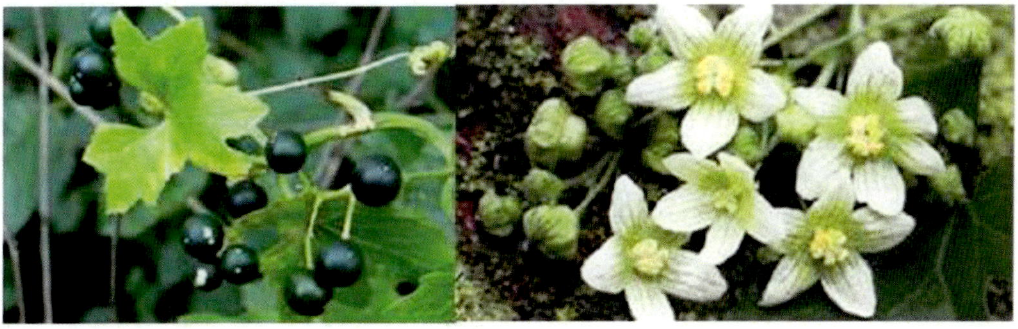

Fig. (7). Bryonia Plant.

2.3.2. Covid 19

Covid 19 is the most devastating pandemic mankind has seen in the last hundreds of years. This viral pandemic is caused by RNA virus and human to human transmission by droplet infection. Its primary target is the respiratory system, leading to symptoms ranging from coryza, cough, sore throat, hoarseness, bronchitis, pneumonia to ARDS and pulmonary fibrosis.

Inflammation and uncontrolled immune response are the pathological events leading to all the complications. Lower respiratory tract is most affected. ACE 2 is the target receptor of COV 2. ACE 2 expression is seen in lung epithelium as inflammation and endothelial injury. Increase in cytokines like IL6, IL 10, which trigger a violent inflammatory response in lung and other organs. Cytokine storm to the lung is a common cause of death.

There are very few effective drugs to control this pathology except steroids. Most of the other drugs used for treatment are found ineffective.

COVID cases, which are mild to moderate were treated with indicated homoeopathic medicines along with a few herbal extracts at Dr. Barve's Clinic in Mumbai as indicated in Table **2**. The drug strength of these hydro alcoholic extracts was 1/10 and was prepared as directed by homeopathic pharmacopeia of India.

Table 2. COVID 19 patients treated with herbal medicines.

S. No	Drug Used	Drug Strength of Ethanolic Extract	Indications	Dose and Repetition	No. of Patients	Results
1	*Aspidosperma quebracho*	1/10	Covid 19 with breathlessness with bilateral pneumonia or ground glass opacities, known as asthmatic, emphysema, O_2 saturation less than 94%	Min. 10 drops with water twice a day to max: 15 drops 4 times	15	Oxygenation and breathlessness improved in 2 days in 70% of patients, out of which 4 cases were on positive pressure O_2
2	*Senega Polygala*	1/10	Old patients with Covid 19, dry cough, rattling mucus, difficult expectoration, dry cough with dyspnoea, viscid mucus, hoarseness, pleural effusion,	Min: 15 drops 3 times with water to max: 20 drops 3 times	18	Senega helped as mucolytic Reduced cough paroxysms in old people esp. with h/o chronic bronchitis, aphonea and hoarseness. Improved in 3-4 days. Helped to clear opacities in lung faster.

(Table 2) cont.....

S. No	Drug Used	Drug Strength of Ethanolic Extract	Indications	Dose and Repetition	No. of Patients	Results
3	*Justicia adhatoda*	1/10	Early stages of Covid to prevent further cytokine storm, cough, coryza, sore throat, acute catarrhal stage	Min. 10 drops 3 times a day with water, Max: 15 drops 4 times a day (excess dose can cause nausea)	24	Reduces catarrhal phase effectively, given in mild cases early in disease phase. Prevents cough leading to breathlessness. Out of 24 only one patient had developed breathlessness

Following drugs were effectively used:

2.3.3. Aspidosperma Quebracho Blanco Tincture [Family Apocynaceae]

This is an evergreen tree that grows in Argentina (Fig. **8**). Tincture is prepared from stem bark. It helps in improving oxygenation, which is an effective remedy for asthma. The tincture given 10-15 drops three to four times a day stimulates the respiratory center. Drug strength is 1/10 in the ethanolic extract [25]. Aspidosperma contains alkaloid, Yohibine and tannins and can be used in bronchitis also since it has anti-inflammatory properties [26].

The lung capacity is increased as it contains alkaloids, Aspidospermine, Aspidosamin, and Quebrachine [27]. Aspidosperma reduces edema, infiltration of cells, and vasodilatation in the lung and thus has anti-inflammatory properties [28]. Aspidosperma is found effective in trials conducted in asthmatic patients [29]. Aspidosperma alkaloids antagonized the spasmodic action of ACTH and histamine on smooth muscle [30].

2.3.4. Justicia Adhatoda Tincture

Justicia adhatoda plant and leaves are used for the preparation of tincture (Fig. **9**). The plant is a rich source of Vitamin C. The active alkaloids are Vasicine, Adhatodine and Vasicinone [31]. The tincture is used for respiratory tract illness, asthma, bronchitis, and cough. It has anti-inflammatory, anti-tussive and mucolytic properties and thus clears mucus secretions. Vascicoline shows good inhibitory activity on replicase RdRP and protease [32]. Vasicine, Vasicol, Vasicinone, Adhatonine have anti-cholinesterase, anti-tussive, and anti-inflammatory activities [33]. Justicia shows anti-bacterial activities against bacteria like *staph aureus, klebsiella,* and *pseudomonas*, which can cause secondary infections of lung. Vasicine and Vasicinone combined together produce broncho dilatory effect in the alcoholic extract [34].

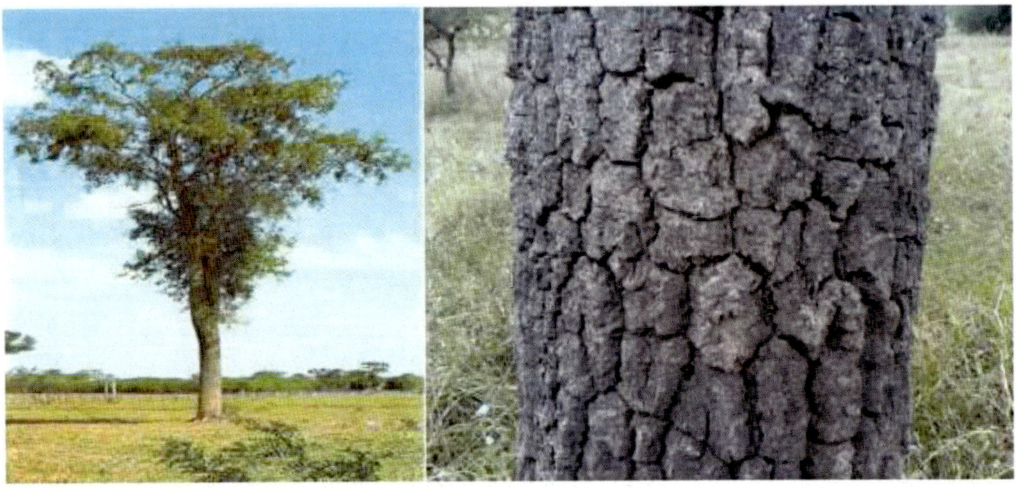

Fig. (8). *Aspidosperma Quebracho Blanco Justicia Adhatoda* Tincture.

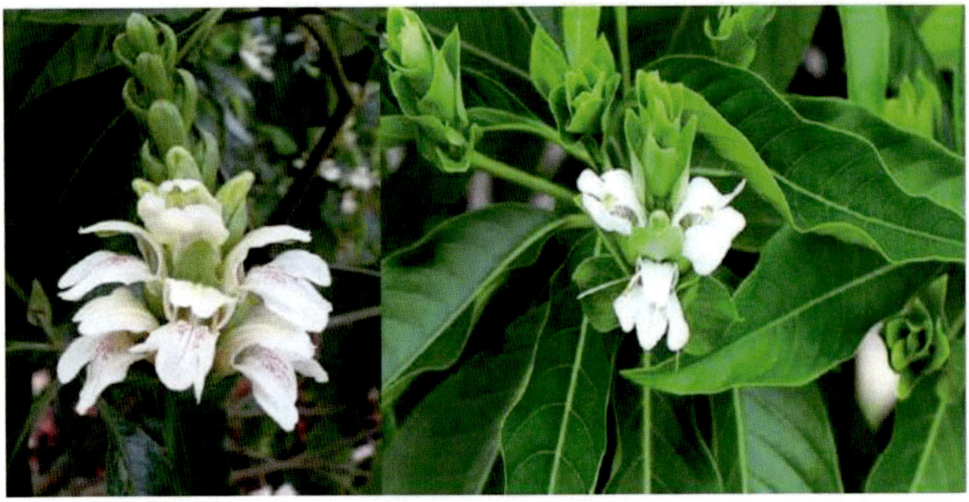

Fig. (9). ***Justicia Adhatoda Senega* Tincture** [Family: *polygalaceae*].

Recent study on Vasicine concludes that Vasicine could be a potential target for the treatment of COVID 19. Vasicine efficacy against corona virus's infection symptoms evaluated in silica screening studies on virus protein ACE 2 receptors, 3CL protease and spike protein SARS HRI motif using PyRx tool and AutoDOC1.5.6 based on PyRx results, vaccine with ACE2 receptors show higher docking affinity score (-7.1 K/cal) repeatedly when compared with other virus proteins [35, 36]. It can be useful in dry cough, hoarseness, suffocative feeling dyspnoea, vomiting, yellowish expectoration, bronchitis and pneumonia [37].

2.3.5. Senega Tincture [Family Polygalaceae]

The flowering plant is perennial and grows in North America and South Canada (Fig. **10**). The common name is snakeroot. The root is used for medicine, as it contains saponins, senegin. sorbitol, sterol and phenolic acid. The *senega* tincture (from roots) is used for dry cough, wheezing, chest congestion, rattling mucus and cough, dyspnoea, aphonea, bronchitis and emphysema [38, 39]. 80% ethanolic extract inhibits inflammatory cytokines IL1B, IL6 when tested in RAW264.7 macrophage cell system [40]. Segega acts as expectorant and expels phelgm, mucollytic action due to saponins in senega, which reduces viscosity of cough [41]. *Senega* has anti-tussive and expectorant activity [42].

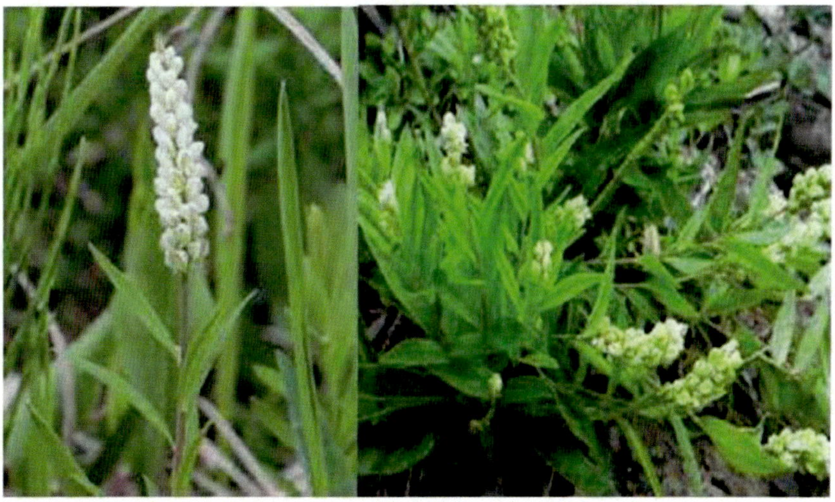

Fig. (10). *Senega Polygala.*

CONCLUDING REMARKS

Herbal medicines and plant extracts are widely used in the treatment of various infectious diseases due to their effectiveness, safety and affordability. Antimicrobial resistance being the major concern in today's modern medicine, the researchers are convinced to go for selecting and standardizing plant treatments since they heal or prevent infectious diseases. There is a need for precisely conducting *in vitro* and *in vivo* studies to target antimicrobial efficacy of plants. The quality of available plant species is limited to a particular geographical area. Because of environmental conditions and pollution, therefore scientific cultivation of medicinal plants is very necessary for the reproducibility of the composition of plant products. On the basis of the increasing resistance of bacteria for standard therapies, the current role of plants could be summarized as treating acute infections, skin or wound infections, and viral diseases, including COVID 19. Rather than using a single extracted alkaloid from the plant, if we use the plant as a whole, as available in nature, the naturally occurring group of alkaloids in the plants have better synergistic action without side effects. Average particle size of homeopathic herbal tinctures used ranged between 2 microns to 34 microns, which helped to deliver medicine to the patients very effectively. The above study shows the effectiveness of plant extracts of *Aegle Folia* and *Holarrhena antidysenterica* in the treatment of gastroenteritis, Aspidosperma, Senega, and Justicia in the treatment of viral bronchitis and cough. Also, for the treatment of viral diseases like dengue, *Eupatorium perfoliatum*, and *Bryonia alba* have shown excellent results. Skin and wound infections with pyogenic bacteria show excellent results (*in vitro* and *in vivo*) using herbal drugs like calendula and echinacea.

ACKNOWLEDGEMENTS

The author (RSC) acknowledges the constant support from Dr. Anushree Lokur, Principal, Ramnarain Ruia Autonomous College, Mumbai, India and also expresses his gratitude to Dr. Barve's Clinic, Mumbai for the clinical results. (RSB) thanks AIMIL Vadodara Laboratory, Vadodara, India and Dr. Pusalkar's laboratory, Sewree, Mumbai, India.

REFERENCES

[1] Munson PL, Muller RA, Beese GR. Principles of Pharmacology Basic Concepts and Clinical Applications. New York: Chapman and Hall 1995; pp. 1-5.

[2] Croteau R, Kutchan TM, Lewis NG. Natural products (secondary metabolites).Biochemistry and Molecular Biology of Plants. USA: American Society of Plant Physiologists 2000; pp. 1250-319.

[3] Efferth T, Koch E. Complex interactions between phytochemicals. The multi-target therapeutic concept of phytotherapy. Curr Drug Targets 2011; 12(1): 122-32. [http://dx.doi.org/10.2174/138945011793591626] [PMID: 20735354]

[4] Heinrich M, Barnes J, Gibbons S, *et al.* Fundamentals of Pharmacognosy and Phytotherapy. London: Elsevier 2004; pp. 161-5.

[5] Milleri M. and Murray J. Diarrhea and constipation, chapter 40, Harrisons's Principles of Internal Medicine, 18th ed., vol.1. p. 308-16.

[6] Rakulini R, Kalaichelvi S. A Review of antidiarrhoeal activity of aegle mar. J Compli and Alternative Medical Res 2019; 7(2): 1-10. [http://dx.doi.org/10.9734/JOCAMR/2019/V7I230095]

[7] Boericke W. Boericke's pocket manual of homeopathy revised ed, 1989, B.Jain publishers, p. 1048.

[8] Sinha S, Sharma A, Reddy PH, Rathi B, Prasad NVSRK, Vashishtha A. Evaluation of phytochem. and pharmacological aspects of Holarrhena Antidysenterica.: a comprehensive review. J Pharm Res 2013; 6(4): 488-92. [http://dx.doi.org/10.1016/j.jopr.2013.04.004]

[9] Nivetha P. Bhuvaragavan PS. Inhibition of multiple SARS-CoV-2 proteins by an antiviral

biomolecule, seselin from Aegle marmelos deciphered using molecular docking analysis. Mol Biol 2020.
[http://dx.doi.org/10.1080/07391102.2021.1955009]

[10] Sunset Western Garden Book. Menlo Park, Calif.: Sunset Pub. Corp. 1995; pp. 606-7.

[11] Stace CA. New Flora of the British Isles. 3rd ed., Cambridge, U.K.: Cambridge University Press 2010.

[12] Ukiya M, Akihisa T, Yasukawa K, Tokuda H, Suzuki T, Kimura Y. Anti-inflammatory, anti-tumo--promoting, and cytotoxic activities of constituents of marigold (Calendula officinalis) flowers. J Nat Prod 2006; 69(12): 1692-6.
[http://dx.doi.org/10.1021/np068016b] [PMID: 17190444]

[13] Yoshikawa M, Murakami T, Kishi A, Kageura T, Matsuda H. Medicinal flowers. III. Marigold. (1): hypoglycemic, gastric emptying inhibitory, and gastroprotective principles and new oleanane-type triterpene oligoglycosides, calendasaponins A, B, C, and D, from Egyptian Calendula officinalis. Chem Pharm Bull (Tokyo) 2001; 49(7): 863-70.
[http://dx.doi.org/10.1248/cpb.49.863] [PMID: 11456093]

[14] Okoh OO, *et al.* The effects of drying on the chemical components of essential oils of *Calendula officinalis* L. Afr J Biotechnol 2008; 7(10): 1500-2.

[15] Leach MJ. Calendula officinalis and Wound Healing: A Systematic Review. Wounds 2008; 20(8): 236-43.
[PMID: 25941793]

[16] Jiménez-Medina E, Garcia-Lora A, Paco L, Algarra I, Collado A, Garrido F. A new extract of the plant *Calendula officinalis* produces a dual *in vitro* effect: cytotoxic anti-tumor activity and lymphocyte activation. BMC Cancer 2006; 6(1): 119.
[http://dx.doi.org/10.1186/1471-2407-6-119] [PMID: 16677386]

[17] Pommier P, Gomez F, Sunyach MP, D'Hombres A, Carrie C, Montbarbon X. Phase III randomized trial of *Calendula officinalis* compared with trolamine for the prevention of acute dermatitis during irradiation for breast cancer. J Clin Oncol 2004; 22(8): 1447-53.
[http://dx.doi.org/10.1200/JCO.2004.07.063] [PMID: 15084618]

[18] Bashir S, Janbaz KH, Jabeen Q, Gilani AH. Studies on spasmogenic and spasmolytic activities of *Calendula officinalis* flowers. Phytother Res 2006; 20(10): 906-10.
[http://dx.doi.org/10.1002/ptr.1980] [PMID: 16906636]

[19] David S, Cunningham R. Echinacea for the prevention and treatment of upper respiratory tract infections: A systematic review and meta-analysis. Complement Ther Med 2019; 44: 18-26.
[http://dx.doi.org/10.1016/j.ctim.2019.03.011] [PMID: 31126553]

[20] Clarence P. Infections caused by arthropod and rhodent born viruses Harrison's Principles of Internal Medicine, Chapter 196, 18th ed., p. 1621-22.

[21] Saeed-ul-Hassan S, Tariq I, Khalid A, Karim S. Comparative Clinical study on the effectiveness of homeopathic combination remedy with standard maintenance therapy. Trop J Pharm Res 2013; 12(5): 767-70.
[http://dx.doi.org/10.4314/tjpr.v12i5.16]

[22] Jatoliya A, John J. Role of Eup. Perf. In cases of dengue fever. European J of Molecular and Clinical Medicine 2020; 7(6): 1794-6.

[23] Phatak SR. Eupatorium Perfoliatum, Materia Medica of Homoeopathic Medicine. I.B.P. 1972; pp. 249-50.

[24] Hensel A, Maas M, Sendker J, *et al.* Eupatorium perfoliatum L.: phytochemistry, traditional use and current applications. J Ethnopharmacol 2011; 138(3): 641-51.
[http://dx.doi.org/10.1016/j.jep.2011.10.002] [PMID: 22004891]

[25] Verma PN. Schwbe's Rare and Clinically Established mother tinctures. 2nd ed. 2006; p. 28.

[26] Fern K. Tropical Plants Database tropical.theferns.info2021. tropical.theferns.info/viewtropical.php?id=Aspidosperma+quebracho-blanco

[27] Horatio CW Jr. Therapeutics of *aspidosperma*. JAMA 1908; L1(19): 1593-4.

[28] De Souza Lima MCJ, *et al*. *Aspidosperma pyrifolium* has anti-inflammatory properties: An Experimental Study in Mice with Peritonitis Induced by Tityusserrulatus Venom or Carrageenan. Int J Mol Sci 2017; 18(11): 2248.
[http://dx.doi.org/10.3390/ijms18112248]

[29] Sukriti, Reddy S, Sharma P, Singh C, *et al*. Bronchial asthma and aspidosperma- A study of 50 patients. TU J. Homeopathy & Med. Sci. 2020; 3(1):24–34.

[30] Banerjee JN, Lewis JJ, Sharp GWG. A preliminary note on the alkaloids of Aspidosperma excelsum Bth. J Pharm Pharmacol 1954; 6(9): 660-2.
[PMID: 13192627]

[31] Dhankar S, Kaur R. Review on justicia adhatoda, Potential Source of Natural Medicine. Afr J Plant Sci 2011; 5(11): 620-7. Corpus ID: 73396926

[32] Bag A, Bag A. Treatment of COVID-19 patients: Justicia adhatoda leaves extract is a strong remedy for COVID-19 – Case report analysis and docking based study. ChemRxiv Cambridge Open Engage 2020.
[http://dx.doi.org/10.26434/chemrxiv.12038604.v1]

[33] Ahmad S, Garg MO, Sanjrani MA, Singh M. A phyto-pharmacological overview on Adhatoda zeylanica Medic. Syn. A. vasica (Linn.). Nees Nat Prod Radiance 2009; 8(5): 549-54. Corpus ID: 27019993.

[34] Baral PK, Roy S, Sultana S. A review article on adhatoda vasicanees: A potential source of bioactive compounds. Int J Dev Res 2018; 8(11): 23874-82.

[35] Thangaraju P, Sudha Ty S, Pasala PK, Hari Ty S, Venkatesan S, Thangaraju E. The Role of Justicia Adhatoda as prophylaxis for COVID-19 - Analysis based on docking study. Infect Disord Drug Targets 2021; 21(8)e160921190441
[http://dx.doi.org/10.2174/1871526521666210119120643] [PMID: 33463480]

[36] Ghosh R, Chakraborty A, Biswas A, Chowdhuri S. Identification of alkaloids from *Justicia adhatoda* as potent SARS CoV-2 main protease inhibitors: An *in silico* perspective. J Mol Struct 2021; 1229129489
[http://dx.doi.org/10.1016/j.molstruc.2020.129489] [PMID: 33100380]

[37] Ghosh SC. Justicia adhatoda, Drugs of Hindustan, 9th ed. 1984, 193–216.

[38] Verma PN, Yadav K. Scwabe's compendium of rare and clinically established mother tinctures, 2nd edition, p.152.

[39] Boericke, William. Pocket Manual of Homoeopathic Materia Medica, 9th ed. Jain Publishers, P.584–85.

[40] Van Q, Nayak BN, Reimer M, Jones PJ, Fulcher RG, Rempel CB. Anti-inflammatory effect of Inonotus obliquus, Polygala senega L., and Viburnum trilobum in a cell screening assay. J Ethnopharmacol 2009; 125(3): 487-93.
[http://dx.doi.org/10.1016/j.jep.2009.06.026] [PMID: 19577624]

[41] Kalra M, Khatak M. Cold and flu: conventional *vs*. Botanical and Nutritional Therapy Int J Drug Dev & Res 2011; 3(1): 314-27.

[42] Gairola S, Gupta V, Bansal P, *et al*. Herbal Antitussives and Expectorants – A Review. Int J Pharm Sci Rev Res 2010; 5(2): 002. Corpus ID: 74727630.

CHAPTER 4

Herbal Medicine: Traditional Approach to Treat Infections

Uttam Singh Baghel[1,2,*], **Nidhi**[2], **Bhanu Pratap Singh**[2] and **Deeksha Singh**[3]

[1] *Gurukul Pharmacy College, Ranpur, Kota – 325003, Rajasthan, India*

[2] *Department of Pharmacy, University of Kota, Kota-324005, Rajasthan, India*

[3] *E. S. I. Hospital, Kota-324005, Rajasthan, India*

Abstract: Infectious diseases are a major cause of morbidity and mortality at a worldwide level. While common cold, encephalitis, meningitis and gastroenteritis are mostly triggered by viruses, cholera, diphtheria, dysentery, tuberculosis, typhoid and pneumonia infections are caused by various bacteria, whereas valley fever, histoplasmosis, candidiasis, ringworm and eye infections are generated by several fungi. Also, ectoparasites like mites, lice, ticks and fleas can be responsible for some infections by attaching to the skin. However, after the onset of COVID-19, which mostly presents as a respiratory disease, a top interest has been put on virus research. Many studies have shown that phytochemicals exert a plethora of biological effects, among them, their antimicrobial action through different mechanisms has been highly underlined. Indeed, they are able to damage the bacterial cell membrane and suppress diverse virulence factors, including inhibition of the activity of various enzymes and toxins and biofilm formation. This chapter summarizes the impact of certain phytochemicals, for example, flavonoids, polyphenols, saponins, steroids, tannins, terpenoids, and alkaloids, as naturally-occurring bioactive compounds present in plants, in several infectious diseases.

Some herbal medicines containing flavonoids form complexes with cell walls of bacteria, protein and extracellular components and are important and effective antimicrobial compounds. Herbal medicines contain terpenoids involved in weakening microorganism cell wall and membranous tissue dissolution, thus inhibiting the growth of infections. Saponins found in herbal medicines cause microbes enzyme leakage from the cell, whereas Steroid in antimicrobial drugs is responsible for liposome leakage from the lipid bilayer membrane. Based on the evidences, the antimicrobial activity of the medicinal plant *Veronica biloba* was found against *E.coli*, *S.aureus*, and *Aspergillus fumigatus* pathogens. The common herbs tarragon and thyme both contain caffeic acid, which is effective against viruses, bacteria, and fungi. Organosulphur compounds such as allicin, isothiocynate and ajoene have shown antibacterial activity against both gram-positive and gram-negative bacteria. Catechins, the most reduced

[*] **Corresponding author Uttam Singh Baghel:** Department of Pharmacy, University of Kota, Kota-324005, Rajasthan, India; Tel: 8528553355; E-mail: uttamsingh1985@gmail.com

Atta-ur-Rahman & Ka Bian (Eds.)

form of the C_3 unit in flavonoid compounds, deserve special mention due to their occurrence in green teas. It was noticed that teas also exerted antimicrobial activity against *Vibrio cholerae*, *S. mutans*, *shigella* and other microorganisms. This chapter focuses on all aspects of infectious diseases and herbal medicines, including chemical constituents and their therapeutic effects.

Keywords: Alkaloids, Antimicrobial, Bacteria, Fungi, Flavoinoids, Saponins, Infectious Diseases, Phytochemicals, Terpenoids, Virus.

1. INTRODUCTION

Out of many several challenges to human health, infectious diseases have a profound effect on the life of humans. All types of infections have different features when compared to other diseases [1]. Primary traits are their unpredictability and probable distinctive effect on the world population, like the pandemic of bubonic-pneumonic plague in the 14th century [2, 3], the influenza pandemic in 1918 [4, 5] and the current pandemic of COVID-19 [6], among others. Infections are generally acute and explicit in nature. The onset of any infectious disease can be instantaneous and distinctive. Furthermore, without any therapeutic intervention, this acute illness shows all or none phenomenon means rapid death and unconstrained recovery. Another unique feature of these infectious diseases is transmission to others. Although the modes of transmission are somewhat less, the most common are inoculation, air and water-mediated transmission. These are well-established and simple to understand, both preclinically and clinically. Majorly, infectious sickness is induced by one pathogen compared to other life-style related diseases induced by multiple co-factors [1]. Infectious diseases can be prevented by general-disease control measures (*e.g.,* hand-washing and sanitization, disinfection by chemicals and vector control) and specific measures (*e.g.,* anti-microbial drug treatment or vaccination).

Although prevention has become more effective, history has depicted that some infectious diseases, especially those that have a wide world impact and for which there is no major non-human source and reservoir, can be eradicated, like poliomyelitis, which has been obliterated from the western hemisphere [7] and smallpox, has been completely removed from the whole world [8]. One more distinctive feature of these pathogens is the marvelous adaptability of replication and mutational changes, which gives them an evolutionary benefit against the aim of their demolition. These adaptations induce the need for the development of new vaccine antigens, *e.g.,* the influenza vaccine, which is updated annually.

2. HERBAL MEDICINAL PLANTS/HERBS COUNTERACTING INFECTIOUS DISEASES

Recently, the popularity of herbal therapy has been increasing day by day, both in developing and developed countries. The research on pharmacological activity, risk/benefit ratio, active phytoconstituents and medicinal values are ongoing worldwide. Research on various aspects of medicinal plants is being executed in Rwanda, Maltese islands, Eastern Africa, Nigeria, Cuba, India, China, European countries, and other countries of the world [9 - 20]. As a precious store of natural medicines, these are attaining much recognition due to their increasing demand and their merits over other treatment systems, including allopathy. These have multiple health advantages and depict much usefulness in complementary systems of medicines as effective therapeutic interventions. These medicinal herbs also play a role in improving and maintaining the general status of health. These medicinal plants provide a cheaper, safer and easily available source of medicines [19, 21, 22].

2.1. Medicinal Plants Used To Treat Bacterial Infections

Several developing as well as developed countries, including India, depend on medicinal plants to treat bacterial infections. These plants include Amla, Heeng, Ashwagandha, Giloy, Arjuna, Turmeric, Ginger, Garlic, Shatawari, Kiwi-fruit, pipali, tea-tree, Neem, Guduchi, Palashlata, Kokilaksha, *etc.* [18 - 20, 23 - 32]. These have many benefits in treating superficial wounds and other ailments caused by bacteria. Some of the best examples are given in Table **1**.

Table 1. Plants/herbs, common name, active phytoconstituents and anti-bacterial activity.

S. No.	Scientific Name	Common Name	Active Phytoconstituents and Mechanism of Action	Extracts Used/ Dose Used	Antibacterial Potential Against	References
1.	***Aloe barbadensis* (*asphodelaceae*)**	Aloevera, Ghrita kumari, Star cactus, Barbados, Guarpatha	**Pyrocatechol:** Act by denaturing proteins and disrupting cell membranes. **Cinnamic acid** inhibits glucose uptake and ATP production in the resting cells of bacteria. **P-coumaric acid:** Increase lag phase of microorganisms. **Ascorbic acid:** Interfering with cell membranes, enzymatic activity and genetic mechanisms.	Aqueous, ethanolic and methanolic extracts	*Pseudomonas, aeruginosa, M. tuberculosis, S. aureus, E. coli, S. typhi, Corynebacterium/ in vitro* study	[33 - 35]

(Table 1) cont.....

S. No.	Scientific Name	Common Name	Active Phytoconstituents and Mechanism of Action	Extracts Used/ Dose Used	Antibacterial Potential Against	References
2.	***Azadirachta indica (Meliaceae)***	Neem	**Azadirachtin, nimbolinin, nimbin, nimbidin, nimbidol, gedunin, salannin, quercitin, β-sitosterol, flavonoids:** Modulation of cell signaling pathways	Aqueous, ethanolic and methanolic extracts from seeds, neem oil/ 125 µg/ml	*Campylobacter jejuni, S. typhi, E. Coli, P. aeruginosa/ in vitro study*	[36 - 39]
3.	***Allium sativum (Amaryllidaceaea)***	Garlic, lasun	**Alliin, allicin, ajoenes, Vinyldithiins, diallyl disulfides, diallyl trisulfides:** trapping the RNA and limiting the speed of RNA	Methanolic and aqueous extracts/ 22.9-32.7 mg/ml	*C. jejuni, S. typhi, E. coli, K. pneumonia/ in vitro study*	[40 - 43]
4.	***Acorus calamus (Acoraceae)***	Calamus, bach, sweet flag	**α-amophene, β-assarone, α-cardinol, α-cedrene, eugenol:** Interrupting the permeability of cell membrane, inhibits the cytochrome c reductase and denatures the cell proteins	Methanolic extract of rhizomes	*S. albus, S. subtilis, S. dysentriae, E. coli/ in vitro study*	[44, 45]
5.	***Andrographis paniculata (Acanthaceae)***	Chirata, Kalmegh	**Andrographolide, de-oxy andrographolide, neo-andrographolide, saponins, tannins and flavonoids:** Inhibition of viral DNA replication, Impairment of proteins, DNA and RNA synthesis	Aqueous, ethanolic and methanolic extract/ 100 µg/ml	*Bacllius cereus, Staphylococcus aureus/ in vitro study*	[46 - 48]
6.	***Annona squamosa (Annonaceae)***	Custard apple, Sitaphal	**Annotemoyin-1 & 2, squamocin, eugenol, farnesol, flavonoids:** Disrupt the peptidoglycan formation, loss of wall's mechanical strength and osmotic lysis	Aqueous, ethanolic, methanolic and acetone extracts of leaves/ 16-51 µg/ml	*S. aureus, B. cereus, B. subtilis, P. aeruginosa/ in vitro study*	[49, 50]
7.	***Actindia macrosperma (Actinidiaceae)***	Wild kiwi, cat ginseng	**1, 2 dimethyllindoline, linalool, linolenic acid methyl ester, alkaloids, polysaccharides, saponins:** Perturbation of bacterial cell wall or cell lysis, inhibition of cytokinesis and bacterial cell proliferation	Hydrodistilled extracted leaf oil/ 0.78-25.5 µl/ml	*S. aureus, B. subtilis, E.coli/ in vitro study*	[51, 52]
8.	***Brassica campestris (Brassicaceae)***	Sarsam, mustard	**Zeaxanthin, glucosinolates, alkaloids, phytosterols:** Protein destabilization produces pores in the cell membrane and causes leakage of intracellular substances	Ethanol, petroleum ether, ethyl acetate extracts of roots	*S. aureus, B. cereus, P. aeruginosa, E. coli/ in vitro study*	[53, 54]

(Table 1) cont.....

S. No.	Scientific Name	Common Name	Active Phytoconstituents and Mechanism of Action	Extracts Used/ Dose Used	Antibacterial Potential Against	References
9.	***Astragalus membranaceus (Fabaceae)***	Astragalus	**Astragalosides, calycosin 7-O-β glucoside, formononetin, liquiritigenin, daidzein, methylnissolin, isomucronulatol:** Alteration of specific cellular components to enhance the changes in bacterial growth properties	Methanolic and ethanolic extracts of roots and leaves/ 8167 μg/ml	*E. coli, S. enteritidis, Shigella sp./ in vitro study*	[55 - 57]
10.	***Calotropis gigantea (Apocynaceae)***	Giant milkweed, Akanda	**Calatropin, giganticin, 19-Nor and 18, 20 epoxy cardinolides, isorhamnetin-3-O-rutinoside, calotropain FI and FII:** Precipitation of proteins by penetrating into the cell wall and cytoplasm of bacteria. Denaturize the enzymes which are involved in the process of germination. These can cause cell lysis by breaking the peptidoglycan bond	Methanolic, chloroform and petroleum ether extracts of root bark/ 1.5-50 mg/ml	*Sarcina lutea, Bacillus megderium, P. aeruginosa, subtilis, Shigella somei/ in vitro study*	[58 - 60]
11.	***Curcuma longa (Zingiberaceae)***	Haldi, Indian saffron, turmeric	**Curcumin, Zingiberene, α and β- turmeron:** Disturbance in membrane permeability and increase fluidity which causes the inhibition of membrane-embedded enzymes, membrane disruption, destruction of the electron transport system and cell wall lysis.	Aqueous, methanolic and ethyl acetate extracts of rhizomes/ 4-28 mg/ml	*Methicillin resistant S. aureus (MRSA), Listeria monocytogenes, Salmonella sp., Shigella sp./ in vitro study*	[61 - 63]
12.	***Camellia sinensis (Theaceae)***	Green tea	**Catechin, epi-catechin:** Irreversibly damages the bacterial cytoplasmic membrane, which reduces the adhesion of bacteria to host cell membrane, so it acts as a potent anti-adhesive agent.	Methanolic and aqueous extracts of dried leaves/ 0.156-0.313 mg/ml	*Shigella sp., Vibrio sp., S. mutans/ in vitro study*	[64 - 66]
13.	***Datura alba (Solanaceae)***	Kaladhatura	**Hyoscyamine, hyoscine, meteloidine:** Not elucidated yet	Ethanolic extracts of leaves	*Staphylococcus sp., Klebsiella sp., E. coli, Pseudomonas sp., Salmonella sp., Vibrio sp.*	[67]

(Table 1) cont.....

S. No.	Scientific Name	Common Name	Active Phytoconstituents and Mechanism of Action	Extracts Used/ Dose Used	Antibacterial Potential Against	References
14.	***Emblica officinalis (Euphorbiaceae)***	Amla, Indian gooseberry	**Ellagic acid, gallic acid, Kaempferol 3 O alpha L (6" methyl rhamnopyronoside, Kaempferol 3 O alpha L (6" ethyl) rhamnopyronoside, high quantity of vitamin C:** Inhibiting adhesion properties of bacteria	Methanolic and aqueous extracts of fresh leaves and fruits/ 5% aqueous solution	*E. coli, K. pneumoniae, K. ozaenae, P. aeruginosa, S. typhi, S. marcescens/ in vitro study*	[68 - 71]
15.	***Cassia angustifolia (Caesalpiniaceae)***	Senna	**Tinnevellin glycoside (I), Isorhamnetin 3-O-beta gentibioside (II), Kaempferol, apigenin-6,8--i-C-glycoside:** Not elucidated yet.	Aqueous extract of seeds and leaves	*S. aureus*	[72]
16.	***Glycyrrhiza glabra (Fabaceae)***	Yashti-maduh, liquorice, sweet wood	**Glycyrrhizic acid, β-Glycyrrhetinic acidglabridin, sterine:** Inhibits synthesis of DNA, RNA and protein	Ethanolic extract of roots and leaves/ 7.6 μg/ml	*B. subtilis, Enterococcus faecailis, M. tuberculosis, E. coli, P. aeruginosa, K. pneumonia/ in vitro study*	[73 - 76]
17.	***Centella asiatica (Apiaceae)***	Gotu kola	**Asiatocoside, α-humulene, β-caryophyllene, bicyclogermacrene, germacrene-B, myrcene, zingibrene:** Weakens the membranous proteins results in the dissolution of the cell wall of bacteria	Ethanolic, aqueous, and chloroform extracts of leaves and roots/ 16 μl/ml	*E. coli, S. aureus, S. albus, Streptococcus pyogenes, pseudomonas aeruginosa, Streptococcus pneumonia/ in vitro study*	[77, 78]
18.	***Foeniculum vulgare (Apiaceae)***	Fennel, Saunf	**Anethole, trans-anethole, essential oils, estragole:** An increase in the electrical conductivity of the cell membrane leads to an increase in the permeability of the cell membrane, further causing the leakage of intracellular ingredients, especially Ca^{2+}, K^{+}, Na^{+} *etc.*	Essential seed oil/ 0.125-0.25 mg/ml	*Bacillus megaterium, S. aureus, E. Coli, Pseudomonas putida, Bacillus pumilus, S. typhi/ in vitro study*	[79 - 81]
19.	***Catharanthus roseus (Apocynaceae)***	Periwinkle, Sadabahar	**Vincristine, Vinblastine, reserpine, serpentine:** Do not show direct antibacterial action but strengthen the immune system of the host	Acetone and ethanolic extracts of whole plant/ 100 mg/ml	*Pseudomonas aeruginosa, E. Coli, S. aureus, S. typhi/ in vitro strudy*	[82 - 85]

(Table 1) cont.....

S. No.	Scientific Name	Common Name	Active Phytoconstituents and Mechanism of Action	Extracts Used/ Dose Used	Antibacterial Potential Against	References
20.	***Mentha piperita (Lamiaceae)***	Peppermint	**Menthol, menthone, methyl acetate, menthofuran, pipperment oil:** Changes in permeability of cell membrane resulting in the leakage of essential intracellular components	Ethanolic, methanolic, ethyl acetate, pet. ether, hexane and chloroform extracts of leaves/ 0.5% v/v solution	*Pseudomonas aeruginosa, E. Coli, S. aureus, B. subtilis, Salmonella typhimurium, B. cereus/ in vitro study*	[86 - 89]
21.	***Ocimum Sanctum (Lamiaceae)***	Tulsi	Oleanolic acid, carvacrol, eugenol-β-caryophyllene, eugenol, rosmarinic acid: Having immunomodulatory effect and act by increasing the level of interferon, interleukin-4 and T-helper cells that can enhance host response to infections	Aqueous and methanolic extracts of fresh leaves and stem/ 80 μg/ml - >2.5 mg/ml	*Methicillin-resistant S. aureus (MRSA), Enterococcus sp., E. Coli, P. aeruginosa, Salmonella sp., Shigella sp./ in vitro study*	[90 - 92]
22.	***Piper longum (Piperaceae)***	Pipali	**Piperine, piperlonguminine, piperlongumine, piplartine:** Obstruction of the respiratory metabolism of bacterial cells	n-Hexane and ethyl acetate extracts of roots/ 12.5 mg/ml	*B. cereus, E. Coli, P. aeruginosa, S. typhi, S. aureus/ in vitro study*	[93 - 95]
23.	***Panax ginseng (Araliaceae)***	Ginseng	Ginsenosides, panaxadiol, panaxatriol: Degrade the cell wall, interact with cellular composition and disrupt the cytoplasmic membrane of bacteria	Aqueous, chloroform and ethanol extracts of roots/ <1 μg/ml	*Staphylococcus aureus, Bacillus subtilis, E. coli, Staphylococcus epidermis/ in vitro study*	[96 - 99]
24.	***Solanum nigrum (Solanaceae)***	Black nightshade	**Solasodine:** Disruption of cell membrane, restricts the cell wall formation, inactivation of microbial adhesins, decreasing the activity of enzymes and blocking of nucleic acid synthesis	Ethanolic and methanolic extracts of stem, leaves, berries and whole plant/ 100 mg/ml	*Bacillus subtilis, E. coli, Klebsiella pneumonia, P. aeruginosa/ in vitro study*	[100 - 102]

2.2. Protozoan Disease

Parasite protozoal diseases are one of the major health issues of the current population worldwide. Some of the biggest ailments that happened due to protozoa and medicinal plants used for their treatment are given in Table **2**.

2.3. Antihelmentic Plants/Herbs

Medicinal plants used to treat anti-helminthic infections are given in Table **3**.

Table 2. Plants/herbs, common name, active phytoconstituents, extract used, and anti-protozoal activity.

S.No.	Scientific Name	Common Name	Active Phytoconstituents	Extracts Used	Anti-Protozoal Potential Against	References
1.	***Cinchona officinalis*** (Rubiaceae)	Cinchona bark	**Quinine:** Prevent the polymerization of the toxic hematin which is formed by the degradation of haemoglobin in erythrocytes to hemozoin. It also blocks the detoxification process developed by the bacteria	Decoction of the bark	*P. falciparum*	[103]
2.	***Aegele marmelos*** (Rutaceae)	Bael	**Tannins:** Inhibition of the adherence of protozoa to the gut epithelium	Unripe or half-ripe fruit/methanol extract of *A. marmelos*	*Rotavirus/ E. coli, Entamoeba histolytica/ in vitro study*	[104, 105]
3.	***Lantana camara*** (verbenaceae)	Lantana, Raimuniya	**Eicosane, squalene, caryophyllene oxide, β- ionone, hexanoic acid, camaric acid, tiglic acid, mixture of lantanilie, β-caryophyllene, lantadene B:** Oxidation of red blood cells and inhibition of the protein synthesis in parasites	Ethyl acetate extract of leaf/ 21.3 μM	*Leishmania mexicana, L. amazonesis/ in vitro study*	[106, 107]

(Table 2) cont.....

S.No.	Scientific Name	Common Name	Active Phytoconstituents	Extracts Used	Anti-Protozoal Potential Against	References
4.	***Momordica charantia*** (Cucurbitaceae)	Bitter melon	**Steroidal saponins (Charantin), momordicine alkaloid, P-insulin, Polypeptide, minerals and aromatic volatile oil:** Inhibition of oxidative phosphorylation and increases the calcium permeability	Aqueous extract of leaves	*Plasmodium falciparum, Entamoeba histolytica*	[108, 109]
5	***Phyllanthus amarus*** (Phyllanthaceae)	Bhumyamalaki	**Saponins, tannins, flavonoids, glycosides, terpenoids, alkaloids:** Blocking the protein synthesis in the malaria parasite	Ethanolic extract of leaves	*P. berghei, Plasmodium falciparum/ in vitro study*	[110, 111]
6.	***Piper nigrum*** (Piperaceae)	Black pepper	**α & β- pinene, myrcene, α-phellandrene, limonene, piperine, α-copaene & caryophyllene:** Act as a neurotoxin and inhibitory action on enzymes	Aqueous extract of dried fruit	*P. falciparum/ in vitro study*	[112, 113]
7.	***Alstonia scholaris*** (Apocynaceae)	Blackboard tree	**Tubotaioine and its oxide, 6,7-seco-angustilobine B, 17-O-acetylechitamine, echitamine, alstonine, villastonine:** Not elucidated yet	Extract of bark	*P. falciparum, Entamoeba histolytica*	[114]

(Table 2) cont.....

S.No.	Scientific Name	Common Name	Active Phytoconstituents	Extracts Used	Anti-Protozoal Potential Against	References
8.	***Berberis aristata*** (Berberidaceae)	Daruhaldhi, Citra	**Berberine, berbamine, colunbamamine, Karachine, Oxyacanthine, oxyberberine, Palmatine, Palmitin, Taxilanine:** Incalation or insertion between the planar bases of DNA	Extract of roots & leaves/ 125-500 µg/ml	*Entamoeba histolytica, Plasmodium berghei/ in vivo study*	115, 116]
9.	***Tinospora cardifolia*** (Memispermaceae)	Amrita	**Tinocardifolin, tinocordifolioside, arabinogalactan, phytoecdysones, ecdysterone, makisterone, berberine, magnoflorine:** Not elucidated yet	Extract of stem	Anti-leishmania	[117]

Table 3. Plants/herbs, common name, active phytoconstituents, extract used and anti-helmentic activity.

S.No.	Scientific Name	Common Name	Active Phyto Constituents	Extracts Used	Antihelmentic Potential Against	References
1.	***Moringa oleifera*** (Moringaceae)	Drumstick	**Saponins, alkaloids, tannins, carbohydrates, steroids, flavonoids:** Stop larval formation and hatching process	Ethanolic extract of the whole herb	*Pheritima Posthuma, Haemonchus contortus/ in vitro study*	[118, 119]

(Table 3) cont.....

S.No.	Scientific Name	Common Name	Active Phyto Constituents	Extracts Used	Antihelmentic Potential Against	References
2.	***Melia azederach*** (Meliaceae)	Persian-lilac	**3-α- benzoate triterpenoid and six other triterpenoids aromatic ester and eight lignans:** a. Connection to free proteins, causes reducing the availability of nutrients, resulting in larval death by starvation. b. Connection to the larval cuticle, rich in glycoproteins, causes larval death.	n- hexane extract of fruits	*Haemonchus contortus/ in vitro study*	[120, 121]
3.	***Semicarpus anacardium*** (Anacardiaceae)	Bhilawa	**Anacardic acid:** Not elucidated yet	Pet. ether, Chloroform, ethanolic and aqueous extract of nuts	*Pheritima Posthuma*	[122]
4.	***Abutilon indicum*** (Malvaceae)	Country mallow	**Abutilon A, asarone, phenolic compounds:** Interfere in the absorption of proteins and lipids, causing damage to the intracellular system. It also breaks energy metabolism and interferes with cell surface glycoproteins, leading to parasite death.	Ethyl acetate extract from leaves	*Eudrillus eugeniae, ascaris lumbricoids/ in vitro*	[123, 124]
5.	***Cucurbita Mexicana*** (cucurbitaceae)	Malabar gourd, kuddu	**Cucurbitin:** Changes in parasite movements, destruction in tegumentine and eggs in reproduction rings of the parasite.	Ethanolic, ethereal, aqueous extract of seeds	*Moniezia expansa, Fasciolopsis buski, Ascaris lumbricoides, Hymenolepis diminuta/ in vivo study*	[125, 126]

(Table 3) cont.....

S.No.	Scientific Name	Common Name	Active Phyto Constituents	Extracts Used	Antihelmentic Potential Against	References
6.	***Carica papaya*** (Carecaceae)	Papaya	**Cysteine proteinases:** Paralysis of parasites	Aqueous extract of seeds	*Trichuris muris, Protospirura muricola/ in vitro study*	[127]
7.	***Tecoma stans*** (Bignoniaceae)	Yellow bell	Indolic compounds: Not elucidated yet	Aqueous, alcoholic and methanolic extract of leaves	*Pheretima Posthuma*	-
8.	***Zingiber zerumbet*** (Zingiberaceae)	Nakachur	**Zerumbone, alpha humulene, humulene epoxide II, caryophyllene oxide and camphene:** Loss of motility and paralysis of parasites occur.	Ethanolic extract of seeds and rhizomes	*Pheretima posthumus*	[128]
9.	***Chenopodium album*** (Amaranthaceae)	Goosefoot, wild spinach	**Tannins, saponins, phytic acid, and alkaloids:** Causes flaccid paralysis of the body muscles.	Methanolic extract of the whole plant	*Haemonchus contortus/ in vitro study*	[129]

2.4. Antiviral Plants/Herbs

Viruses are one of the major threats to both the human population and animals worldwide. They go inside the living body and interfere with the body's metabolism and make huge copies of their genomes. It is very difficult to control these viruses with the help of recently available anti-viral drugs. Therefore we need some medicinal plants/herbs to tackle viral infections. Some of the best examples of anti-viral medicinal plants along with their active phytoconstituents, are mentioned in Table **4**.

Table 4. Plants/herbs, common name, active phytoconstituents, extract used and anti-viral activity.

S.No.	Scientific Name	Common Name	Active Phytoconstituents	Extracts Used	Anti-viral Potential Against	References
1.	***Echinacea purpurea*** (Asteraceae)	Purple coneflower	**Alkamides, caffeic acid derivatives and polysaccharides:** Inhibits haemagglutination activity of the virus and consequently block the entry of the virus into cells	n-hexane extract of aerial parts & roots	*Influenza, Herpes simplex virus/ in vitro study*	[130 - 132]
2.	***Phyllanthus urinaria*** (Phyllanthaceae)	Leaf flower	**Hippomanin A:** Reduced HBV DNA level and inhibits HBV replication and expression	Acetone extract	*Herpes simplex type 2 virus, Hepatitis B virus*	[133, 134]
3.	***Allium sativum*** (Amaryllidaceae)	Garlic, Lasun	**Allicin, allyl methyl thiosulfinate, ajoene:** Interference with virus adsorption and penetration	Fresh extract of garlic, Oil	*Herpes simplex virus*	[135]
4.	***Bostrychia montagmei*** (Rhodomelaceae)	Red alga	**Sulphated polysaccharides:** Inhibits the virus replication	Aqueous extract	*Herpes simplex virus*	[136]
5.	***Cocos nucifera*** (Arecaceae)	Coconut palm	**Catechin, epicatechin, B- type procyanidins:** Interference with virus adsorption and penetration	Water extract of husk fibre	*Herpes simplex virus*	[137]
6.	***Hamamelis virginiana*** (Hamamelidaceae)	Witch hazel	**Oligomeric to polymeric proanthocyanidins:** N/A	Hydroalcoholic extract	*Herpes simplex virus*	[138]
7.	***Myrica rubra*** (myricaceae)	Chinese bayberry	**Tannins (prodelphindin B-2,3,3',di-O- gallate):** Inhibits the viral attachment with cell	Extract of bark	*Herpes simplex virus*	[139]
8.	***Agastache rugosa*** (Lamiaceae)	Mints	**Rosmarinic acid**: N/A	Aqueous & methanolic extract of roots	*Human immunodeficiency virus (HIV)*	[140]
9.	***Caryophyllum brasilence*** (Guttiferae)	Brazil beauty leaf	**Apetalic acid, calanolides B&C**: N/A	n-hexane extract of leaves	*Human immunodeficiency virus (HIV)*	[141]
10.	***Gelonium multiforum*** (Euphorbiaceae)	False lime, Linau –hantu	**GAP-31 protein**: Interaction with ribosomes in infected cells and depresses viral protein synthesis	Protein extract	*Human immunodeficiency virus (HIV)*	[142]
11.	***Kadsura heteroclite*** (Schisandraceae)	N/A	**Triterpenoid and lignans (Dibenzocyclooctadiene-type):** N/A	Extract of stems	*Human immunodeficiency virus (HIV)*	[143]
12.	***Ricinus communis*** (Euphorbiaceae)	Castor bean	**Lectin:** Inhibits reverse transcriptase and N-glycohydrolases	Extract of leaves	*Human immunodeficiency virus (HIV)*	[144]

(Table 4) cont.....

S.No.	Scientific Name	Common Name	Active Phytoconstituents	Extracts Used	Anti-viral Potential Against	References
13.	***Aronia melanocarpa*** (Rosaceae)	Black chokeberry	**Anthocyanins:** N/A	Fruit juice	*Influenza virus*	[145]
14.	***Narcissus tazetta*** (Amaryllidaceae)	Chinese sacred lily	**Narcissus tazetta lectin:** N/A	Bulbs	*Influenza, respiratory syncytial virus*	[146]
15.	***Phyllanthus urinaria*** (Phyllanthaceae)	Leaf flower	**Methyl ester dehydrochebulic acid and methyl brevifolin carboxylate:** N/A	Leaves	*Hepatitis B virus*	[147]
16.	***Embelia schimperi*** (Myrsinaceae)	N/A	**Benzoquinones (embelin I and 5-o-methyl embelin II):** Inhibits HCV proteases	Methanol extract	*Hepatitis C virus*	[148]
17.	***Schefflera heptaphylla*** (Araliaceae)	N/A	**3,4,di-O-caffeoylquinic acid and 3,5-di-O-caffeoylquinic acid:** Inhibition of viral cell fusion	N/A	*Respiratory syntical virus*	[149]

CONCLUSION

Fighting bacterial, protozoal, helminthic and viral infections is the routine process of human and animal life. New therapeutic approaches are coming with advancements in medical science but continuously rising MDR microorganisms. A decline in the efficiency of allopathic medicines against resistant species has created a demand for healthcare professionals to reconsider the traditional methods of treatment. The use of traditional medicinal plants/herbs is quite safe and economical in comparison to modern allopathic approaches. Hence, the present chapter tried to collect as much as possible information from nature's treasures in order to achieve good health and provide desired protection against various pathogens and ailments.

REFERENCES

[1] Fauci AS, Morens DM. The perpetual challenge of infectious diseases. N Engl J Med 2012; 366(5): 454-61.
[http://dx.doi.org/10.1056/NEJMra1108296] [PMID: 22296079]

[2] Hecker JFC. Der schwarze Tod im vierzehnten Jahrhundert. Berlin: Friedrich August Herbig 1832.

[3] Morens DM, Folkers GK, Fauci AS. Emerging infections: a perpetual challenge. Lancet Infect Dis 2008; 8(11): 710-9.
[http://dx.doi.org/10.1016/S1473-3099(08)70256-1] [PMID: 18992407]

[4] Jordan EO. Epidemic influenza: a survey. Chicago: American Medical Association 1927; pp. 60-97.

[5] Morens DM, Fauci AS. The 1918 influenza pandemic: insights for the 21st century. J Infect Dis 2007; 195(7): 1018-28.
[http://dx.doi.org/10.1086/511989] [PMID: 17330793]

[6] Logeswari J, Shankar S, Biswas PG, Muninathan N. Role of Medicinal Plants in the Prevention of Covid-19 Pandemic. Med-Leg Update 2020; 20(4): 2303-6.

[7] de Quadros CA, Andrus JK, Olive JM, Guerra de Macedo C, Henderson DA. Polio eradication from the Western Hemisphere. Annu Rev Public Health 1992; 13(1): 239-52. [http://dx.doi.org/10.1146/annurev.pu.13.050192.001323] [PMID: 1599587]

[8] Fenner F. Smallpox: emergence, global spread, and eradication. Hist Philos Life Sci 1993; 15(3): 397-420. [PMID: 7529932]

[9] Odebiyi OO, Sofowora EA. Phytochemical screening of Nigerian medicinal plants II. Lloydia 1978; 41(3): 234-46. [PMID: 672462]

[10] Lanfranco G. Popular use of medicinal plants in the Maltese Islands. Insula (Madrid) 1992; 1: 34-5.

[11] Vlietinck AJ, Van Hoof L, Totté J, *et al.* Screening of hundred Rwandese medicinal plants for antimicrobial and antiviral properties. J Ethnopharmacol 1995; 46(1): 31-47. [http://dx.doi.org/10.1016/0378-8741(95)01226-4] [PMID: 7475121]

[12] Fabry W, Okemo PO, Ansorg R. Antibacterial activity of East African medicinal plants. J Ethnopharmacol 1998; 60(1): 79-84. [http://dx.doi.org/10.1016/S0378-8741(97)00128-1] [PMID: 9533435]

[13] Barrett B, Kiefer D, Rabago D. Assessing the risks and benefits of herbal medicine: an overview of scientific evidence. Altern Ther Health Med 1999; 5(4): 40-9. [PMID: 10394673]

[14] Bhatt DC, Mitaliya KD, Mehta SK, Joshi PN. Notes on some ethnomedicinal plants of Paccham Hills of Kachh district, Gujarat. Ethnobotany 2002; 14: 34-5.

[15] Cano JH, Volpato G. Herbal mixtures in the traditional medicine of eastern Cuba. J Ethnopharmacol 2004; 90(2-3): 293-316. [http://dx.doi.org/10.1016/j.jep.2003.10.012] [PMID: 15013195]

[16] Arora DS, Kaur GJ. Antibacterial activity of some Indian medicinal plants. J Nat Med 2007; 61(3): 313-7. [http://dx.doi.org/10.1007/s11418-007-0137-8]

[17] Basha SK, Sudarshanam G. Multiple herbal therapy-antimicrobial activity of wound healing paste (Pasuru) used by Sugali tribes of Yerramalais of Kurnool district. Andhra Pradesh, India. Int J Pharm Tech Res 2011; 3: 1238-41.

[18] Mizaei-Aghsaghali A. Importance ofmedical herbs in animal feeding: A review. Ann Biol Res 2012; 3: 918-23. Corpus ID: 17698093.

[19] Mahima A, Rahal A, Deb R, *et al.* Immunomodulatory and therapeutic potentials of herbal, traditional/indigenous and ethnoveterinary medicines. Pak J Biol Sci 2012; 15(16): 754-74. [http://dx.doi.org/10.3923/pjbs.2012.754.774] [PMID: 24175417]

[20] Midrarullah SH, Attaullah S. Sikandar and Ali MS. Traditional uses of medicinal plants for the treatment of livestock ailments in Udigram Swat, Khyber Pakhtunkhwa, Pakistan. Res Opin Anim Vet Sci 2014; 4: 138-41.

[21] Dhar RS, Verma V, Suri KA, *et al.* Phytochemical and genetic analysis in selected chemotypes of Withania somnifera. Phytochemistry 2006; 67(20): 2269-76. [http://dx.doi.org/10.1016/j.phytochem.2006.07.014] [PMID: 16956635]

[22] Kumar A, Kaul MK, Bhan MK, Khanna PK, Suri KA. Morphological and chemical variation in 25 collections of the Indian medicinal plant, Withania somnifera (L.) Dunal (Solanaceae). Genet Resour Crop Evol 2007; 54(3): 655-60. [http://dx.doi.org/10.1007/s10722-006-9129-x]

[23] Archana SJ, Paul R, Tiwari A. Indian medicinal plants: A rich source of natural immune modulator. Int J Pharmacol 2011; 198-205. [http://dx.doi.org/10.3923/ijp.2011.198.205]

[24] Umashanker M, Shruti S. Traditional Indian herbal medicine used as antipyretic, antiulcer, anti-diabetic and anticancer: A review. Int J Res Pharm Chem 2011; 1: 1152-9. Corpus ID: 74070576

[25] Dhama K, Mani S, Chakraborty S, *et al.* Herbal remedies to combat cancers in humans and animals: A review. Int J Curr Res 2013; 5: 1908-19.

[26] Kumar HB, Singh TK. Goswami, Rawat M. Use of neem preparations for the treatment of end ometrit is in cows. Adv Anim Vet Sci 2013; 1: 194-6. b

[27] Kumar A, Rahal A, Chakraborty S, Tiwari R, Latheef SK, Dhama K. *Ocimum sanctum* (Tulsi): A miracle herb and boon to medical science-A review. Int J Agron Plant Prod 2013; 4: 1580-9. Corpus ID: 85674370.

[28] Yakout SM, Abd-Alrahman SH, Mostafa A, Salem-Bekhit MM. Antimicrobial effect of seed ethanolic extract of Coriander. J Pure Appl Microbiol 2013; 7: 459-63.

[29] Tiwari R, Latchumikanthan A. Yadav RK and Dhama K. Herbal and traditional botanical medicines for safeguarding animal and human health. Livestock Line 2012; 6: 29-33.

[30] Tiwari RS, Chakraborty S, Dhama K. Miracle of herbs in antibiotic resistant wounds and skin infections: Treasure of nature-are view/perspective. Pharma Sci Monitor 2013; 4: 214-48.

[31] Tiwari R, Chakrabort S, Saminathan M, Dhama K, Singh SV. Ashwagandha *(Withania somnifera):* Role in safeguarding health, immunomodulatory effects, combating infections and therapeutic applications: A review. J Biol Sci (Faisalabad, Pak) 2014; 14(2): 77-94. d [http://dx.doi.org/10.3923/jbs.2014.77.94]

[32] Tiwari R, Verma AK, Chakrabort S, Dhama K, Singh SV. Neem *(Azadirachta indica)* and its potential for safeguarding health of animals and humans: A review. J Biol Sci (Faisalabad, Pak) 2014; 14(2): 110-23. e [http://dx.doi.org/10.3923/jbs.2014.110.123]

[33] Grace OM, Simmonds MSJ, Smith GF, van Wyk AE. Therapeutic uses of *Aloe* L. (Asphodelaceae) in southern Africa. J Ethnopharmacol 2008; 119(3): 604-14. [http://dx.doi.org/10.1016/j.jep.2008.07.002] [PMID: 18682283]

[34] Alemdar S, Agaoglu S. Investigation of *in vitro* antimicrobial activity of *Aloe vera* juice. J Anim Vet Adv 2009; 8: 99-102.

[35] Lawrence R, Tripathi P, Jeyakumar E. Jeyakumar. Isolation, purification and evaluation of antibacterial agents from *aloe vera.* Braz J Microbiol 2009; 40(4): 906-15. [http://dx.doi.org/10.1590/S1517-83822009000400023] [PMID: 24031440]

[36] Jahan T, Begum ZA, Sultana S. Effect of neem oil on somepathogenic bacteria. Bangladesh J Pharmacol 2007; 2: l-72. [http://dx.doi.org/10.3329/BJP.V2I2.573]

[37] El-Mahmood AM, Ogbonna OB. The antibacterial activity of *Azadarichta indica* (neem) seeds extracts against bacterial pathogens associated with eye and ear infections. J Med Plants Res 2010; 14: 1414-21. [http://dx.doi.org/10.5897/JMPR09.169]

[38] Koona S, Budida S. Antibacterial potential of the extracts of the leaves of *Azadirachta indica* Linn. Not Sci Biol 2011; 3(1): 65-9. [http://dx.doi.org/10.15835/nsb315470]

[39] Parashar G, Sutar N, Sanap S. Antibacterial activity of mixture of leaf extracts of neem (*azadirachta indica* linn.) And tantani (*lantana camara*). IJPSR 2018; 9: 2545-9.

[40] Venugopal PV, Venugopal TV. Antidermatophytic activity of garlic (*Allium sativum*) *in vitro*. Int J Dermatol 1995; 34(4): 278-9.
[http://dx.doi.org/10.1111/j.1365-4362.1995.tb01597.x] [PMID: 7790146]

[41] Agarwal KC. Therapeutic actions of garlic constituents. Med Res Rev 1996; 16(1): 111-24.
[http://dx.doi.org/10.1002/(SICI)1098-1128(199601)16:1<111::AID-MED4>3.0.CO;2-5] [PMID: 8788216]

[42] Karuppiah P, Rajaram S. Antibacterial effect of *Allium sativum* cloves *and Zingiber officinale* rhizomes against multiple-drug resistant clinical pathogens. Asian Pac J Trop Biomed 2012; 2(8): 597-601.
[http://dx.doi.org/10.1016/S2221-1691(12)60104-X] [PMID: 23569978]

[43] Mozaffari Nejad AS, Shabani S, Bayat M, Hosseini SE. Antibacterial Effect of Garlic Aqueous Extract on *Staphylococcus aureus* in Hamburger. Jundishapur J Microbiol 2014; 7(11)e13134.
[http://dx.doi.org/10.5812/jjm.13134] [PMID: 25774277]

[44] Phongpaichit S, Pujenjob N, Rukachaisirikul V, Ongsakul M. Antimicrobial activities of the crude methanol extract of *Acorus calamus* Linn. Songklanakarin J Sci Technol 2005; 27: 517-23. Corpus ID: 52237026.

[45] Rita WS, Swantara MD. PrimandaniUtami GA. Proceedings of the 2nd International Conference on Biosciences and Medical Engineering (ICBME 2019). AIP Conf. Proc.2155.
[http://dx.doi.org/10.1063/1.5125558]

[46] Mishra US, Mishra A, Kumari R, Murthy PN, Naik BS. Antibacterial activity of ethanol extract of *Andrographis paniculata.* Indian J Pharm Sci 2009; 71(4): 436-8.
[http://dx.doi.org/10.4103/0250-474X.57294] [PMID: 20502551]

[47] Malahubban M, Alimon AR, Sazili AQ, Fakurazi S, Zakry FA. Phytochemical analysis of *Andrographis paniculata and Orthosiphon stamineus* leaf extracts for their antibacterial and antioxidant potential. Trop Biomed 2013; 30(3): 467-80.
[PMID: 24189677]

[48] Banerjee M, Parai D, Chattopadhyay S, Mukherjee SK. Andrographolide: antibacterial activity against common bacteria of human health concern and possible mechanism of action. Folia Microbiol (Praha) 2017; 62(3): 237-44.
[http://dx.doi.org/10.1007/s12223-017-0496-9] [PMID: 28097636]

[49] El-Chaghaby GA, Ahmad AF, Ramis ES. Evaluation of the antioxidant and antibacterial properties of various solvents extracts of *Annona squamosa* L. leaves. Arab J Chem 2014; 7(2): 227-33.
[http://dx.doi.org/10.1016/j.arabjc.2011.06.019]

[50] Dholvitayakhun A, Trachoo N, Narkkong N, Cushnie TPT. Using scanning and transmission electron microscopy to investigate the antibacterial mechanism of action of the medicinal plant Annona squamosa Linn. J Herb Med 2017; 7: 31-6.
[http://dx.doi.org/10.1016/j.hermed.2016.10.003]

[51] Lu Y, Zhao YP, Wang ZC, Chen SY, Fu CX. Composition and antimicrobial activity of the essential oil of *Actinidia macrosperma* from China. Nat Prod Res 2007; 21(3): 227-33.
[http://dx.doi.org/10.1080/14786410601132311] [PMID: 17365713]

[52] Zhao YP, Fu CX. Preliminary evaluation of antimicrobial and cytotoxic activities of extracts from *Actinidia macrosperma.* Adv Mat Res 2012; 455: 1200-3.
[http://dx.doi.org/10.4028/www.scientific.net/AMR.455-456.1200]

[53] Agrawal MK, Rathore D, Goyal S, Varma A, Varma A. Antibacterial efficacy of *Brassica campestris* root, stem and leaves extracts. Int J Adv Res (Indore) 2013; 1: 131-5.

[54] Khameneh B, Iranshahy M, Soheili V, Fazly Bazzaz BS. Review on plant antimicrobials: a mechanistic viewpoint. Antimicrob Resist Infect Control 2019; 8(1): 118.
[http://dx.doi.org/10.1186/s13756-019-0559-6] [PMID: 31346459]

[55] Balachandar S, Jagadeeswari M, Dhanabalan R, Meenachi M. Antimicrobial activity of *Astragalus membranaceus* against diarrheal bacterial pathogens. Int J Pharm 2012; 2: 416-8.

[56] Teyeb H, Zanina N, Neffati M, Douki W, Najjar MF. Cytotoxic and antibacterial activities of leaf extracts of Astragalus gombiformis Pomel (Fabaceae) growing wild in Tunisia. Turk J Biol 2012; 36: 53-8.
[http://dx.doi.org/10.3906/biy-1010-131]

[57] Lai W, Cock IE, Cheesman MJ. Interactive Antimicrobial Profiles of Astragalus membranaceus (Fisch.) Bunge Extracts and Conventional Antibiotics against Pathogenic and Non-pathogenic Gastrointestinal Bacteria. Pharmacogn Commun 2018; 8(4): 158-64.
[http://dx.doi.org/10.5530/pc.2018.4.33]

[58] Alam MA, Habib MR, Nikkon R, Rahman M, Karim MR. Antimicrobial Activity of Akanda *(Calotrop is gigantean* L.) on some pathogenic bacteria. Bangladesh J Sci Ind Res 1970; 43(3): 397-404.
[http://dx.doi.org/10.3329/bjsir.v43i3.1156]

[59] Anitha M, Hema Priya J, Bhaghyraj A. Joeal. Efficacy of anti-bacterial activity of *Calotro pis gigantean* latex extract-an *in-vitro* study. Int J Recent Sci Res 2014; 5: 113-7.

[60] Hasballah K. Antibacterial Activity of Methanol Extract of Calotropis gigantean Flowers from Aceh. Proceedings of the 2nd Syiah Kuala International Conference on Medicine and Health Sciences - SKIC-MHS, Banda Aceh, Indonesia 2018; 196-200.

[61] Kim KJ, Yu HH, Cha JD, Seo SJ, Choi NY, You YO. Antibacterial activity of *Curcuma longa* L. against methicillin-resistant *Staphylococcus aureus.* Phytother Res 2005; 19(7): 599-604.
[http://dx.doi.org/10.1002/ptr.1660] [PMID: 16161063]

[62] Fazreen N. Determination of antibacterial activity of *Curcuma longa* against selected food poisoning causing bacteria. Proceeding of the Malaysian Science Technology Congress. November 19-21, 2012.

[63] Pundir RK, Jain P. Comparative studies on the antimicrobial activity of Black pepper (piper nigrum) and Turmeric (curcuma longa) extracts. Int J Appl Boil Pharm 2010; 1: 492-501. Corpus ID: 7732494

[64] Matsubara S, Shibata H, Ishikawa F, *et al.* Suppression of *Helicobacter pylori-induced* gastritis by green tea extract in Mongolian gerbils. Biochem Biophys Res Commun 2003; 310(3): 715-9.
[http://dx.doi.org/10.1016/j.bbrc.2003.09.066] [PMID: 14550260]

[65] Gonbad RA, Afzan A, Karimi E, Sinniah UR, Swamy MK. Phytoconstituents and antioxidant properties among commercial tea (Camellia sinensis L.) clones of Iran. Electron J Biotechnol 2015; 18(6): 433-8.
[http://dx.doi.org/10.1016/j.ejbt.2015.08.007]

[66] Sharma A, Gupta S, Sarethy IP, Dang S, Gabrani R. Green tea extract: possible mechanism and antibacterial activity on skin pathogens. Food Chem 2012; 135(2): 672-5.
[http://dx.doi.org/10.1016/j.foodchem.2012.04.143] [PMID: 22868144]

[67] Qureshi MN, Siddique M, Kanwal IR, Kanwal F. Analytical characterization of fatty acids composition of *Datura alba* seed oil by gas chromatograph mass spectrometry. J Chin Chem Soc (Taipei) 2011; 58(2): 236-40.
[http://dx.doi.org/10.1002/jccs.201190082]

[68] Saeed S, Tariq P. Antibacterial activities of *Emblica officinalis and Coriandrum sativum* against Gram negative urinary pathogens. Pak J Pharm Sci 2007; 20(1): 32-5.
[PMID: 17337425]

[69] Vijayalakshmi S, Arunkumar V, Anju D, Gunasundari P, Moorthy P, Chandrasekharan AK. Comparative antimicrobial activities of *Emblica officinalis* and *Ocimum sanctum.* Anc Sci Life 2007; 27(2): 1-6.
[PMID: 22557261]

[70] Jain R, Pandey R, Mahant RN, Rathore DS. A review on medical importance of *Emblica officinalis*. IJPSR 2015; 6(1): 72-84.

[71] Dasaroju S, Gottumukkala KM. Current Trends in the Research of *Emblica officinalis* (Amla): A Pharmacological Perspective. Int J Pharm Sci Rev Res 2014; 24: 150-9. Corpus ID: 73810493

[72] Roopashree TS, Dang R, Shobha Rani RH, Narendra C. Antibacterial activity of antipsoriatic herbs: *Cassia tora, Momordica charantia and Calendula officinalis*. Int J Appl Res Nat Prod 2008; 1: 20-8. Corpus ID: 216040846

[73] Irani MM, Sarmadi F, Bernard GH. Pour Eand Bazarnov HS. Leaves antimicrobial activity of *Glycyrrhizaglabra* L. Iran J Pharm Res 2010; 9: 425-8.
[PMID: 24381608]

[74] Sedighinia F, Safipour Afshar A, Soleimanpour S, Zarif R, Asili J, Ghazvini K. Antibacterial activity of *Glycyrrhiza glabra* against oral pathogens: an *in vitro* study. Avicenna J Phytomed 2012; 2(3): 118-24.
[PMID: 25050240]

[75] Kaur R, Kaur H, Dhindsa AS. Glycrrhiza Glabra: A Phtopharmacological review. IJPSR 2013; 4(7): 2470-7.

[76] Kim HK, Park Y, Kim HN, *et al.* lee DG, Hahm KS. Antimicrobial mechanism of β-glycyrrhetinic acid isolated from licorice, *Glycyrrhizaglabra*. Biotechnol Lett 2002; 24(22): 1899-902.
[http://dx.doi.org/10.1023/A:1020900124997]

[77] Yusuf Nasu M, Restuati M, Shafwan S A, Pratiwi N, Setya Dini D, Diningrat DS. Antimicrobial Activities of *Centella asiatica* Leaf and Root Extracts on Selected Pathogenic Micro-organisms. J Med Sci (Faisalabad, Pak) 2018; 18(4): 198-204.
[http://dx.doi.org/10.3923/jms.2018.198.204]

[78] Pitinidhipat N, Yasurin P. Antibacterial Activity of Chrysanthemum indicum, Centella asiatica and Andrographis paniculata against Bacillus cereus and Listeria monocytogenes under Osmotic Stress. AU JT 2012; 15: 239-45.

[79] Ruberto G, Baratta MT, Deans SG, Dorman HJD. Antioxidant and antimicrobial activity of *Foeniculum vulgare and Crithmum maritimum* essential oils. Planta Med 2000; 66(8): 687-93.
[http://dx.doi.org/10.1055/s-2000-9773] [PMID: 11199122]

[80] Diao WR, Hu QP, Zhang H, Xu JG. Chemical composition, antibacterial activity and mechanism of action of essential oil from seeds of fennel (Foeniculum vulgare Mill.). Food Control 2014; 35(1): 109-16.
[http://dx.doi.org/10.1016/j.foodcont.2013.06.056]

[81] AbduRahim SA, Elamin BEK, Bashir AAA, Almagboul AZ. *In Vitro* Test Of Antimicrobial Activity Of Foeniculum Vulgare Mill. (Fennel) Essential Oil. J. Multidiscp. Engg. Sci. Stud. 2017; 3(4): 1609-14.

[82] Goyal P, Khanna A, Chauhan A, Chauhan G, Kaushik P. *In vitro* evaluation of crude extracts of *Catharanthus roseus* for potential antibacterial activity. Int J Green Pharm 2008; 2(3): 176-81.
[http://dx.doi.org/10.4103/0973-8258.42739]

[83] Govindasamy C, Srinivasan R. *In vitro* antibacterial activity and phytochemical analysis of Catharanthus roseus (Linn.) G. Don. Asian Pac J Trop Biomed 2012; 2(1): S155-8.
[http://dx.doi.org/10.1016/S2221-1691(12)60148-8]

[84] Wagay SA, Dwivedi SD, Sharma M, Tripathi J, Ahmad M. Antimicrobial Activity of Catharanthus Roseus. Chem Mat Res 2013; 3(9): 61-4.

[85] Patil PJ, Ghosh J. Antimicrobial Activity of Catharanthus roseus – A Detailed Study. Br J Pharmacol 2010; 1: 40-4.

[86] Gentry EJ, Jampani HB, Keshavarz-Shokri A, *et al.* Antitubercular natural products: berberine from

the roots of commercial Hydrastis canadensis powder. Isolation of inactive 8-oxotetrahydrothalifendine, canadine, beta-hydrastine, and two new quinic acid esters, hycandinic acid esters-1 and -2. J Nat Prod 1998; 61(10): 1187-93.
[http://dx.doi.org/10.1021/np9701889] [PMID: 9784149]

[87] Sujana P, Sridhar TM, Josthna P, Naidu CV. Antibacterial activity and phytochemical analysis of *Menthapiperita* L. (Peppermint)-animportant multipurpose medicinal plant. Am J Plant Sci 2013; 4(1): 77-83.
[http://dx.doi.org/10.4236/ajps.2013.41012]

[88] Marwa C, Fikri-Benbrahim K, Ou-Yahia D, Farah A. African peppermint (*Mentha piperita*) from Morocco: Chemical composition and antimicrobial properties of essential oil. J Adv Pharm Technol Res 2017; 8(3): 86-90.
[PMID: 28795021]

[89] Singh R, Shushni MAM, Belkheir A. Antibacterial and antioxidant activities of Mentha piperita L. Arab J Chem 2015; 8(3): 322-8.
[http://dx.doi.org/10.1016/j.arabjc.2011.01.019]

[90] Kumar A, Rahal A, Chakraborty S, Tiwari R, Latheef SK, Dhama K. *Ocimum sanctum* (Tulsi): A miracle herb and boon to medical science-A review. Int J Agron Plant Prod 2013; 4: 1580-9. c

[91] Saharkhiz MJ, Kamyab AA, Kazerani NK, Zomorodian K, Pakshir K, Rahimi MJ. Chemical Compositions and Antimicrobial Activities f Ocimum sanctum L. Essential Oils at Different harvest Stages. Jundishapur J Microbiol 2015; 18(1): 1-20.
[PMID: 25763132]

[92] Mallikarjun S, Rao A, Rajesh G, Shenoy R, Pai M. Antimicrobial efficacy of Tulsi leaf (*Ocimum sanctum*) extract on periodontal pathogens: An *in vitro* study. J Indian Soc Periodontol 2016; 20(2): 145-50.
[PMID: 27143825]

[93] Srinivasa Reddy P, Jamil K, Madhusudhan P, Anjani G, Das B. Antibacterial activity of isolates from *Piper longum and Taxus baccata.* Pharm Biol 2001; 39(3): 236-8.
[http://dx.doi.org/10.1076/phbi.39.3.236.5926]

[94] Singh C, Singh SK, Nath G, Rai NP. Anti-mycobacterial activity of P*iper longum* L. fruit extracts against multi drug resistant *Mycobacterium* spp. Int J Phytomed 2011; 3: 353-61.

[95] Zou L, Hu Y-Y, Chen WX. Antibacterial mechanism and activities of black pepper chloroform extract. J Food Sci Technol 2015; 52(12): 8196-203.
[http://dx.doi.org/10.1007/s13197-015-1914-0] [PMID: 26604394]

[96] Lee JH, Shim JS, Lee JS, Kim MK, Chung MS, Kim KH. Pectin-like acidic polysaccharide from *Panax ginseng* with selective antiadhesive activity against pathogenic bacteria. Carbohydr Res 2006; 341(9): 1154-63.
[http://dx.doi.org/10.1016/j.carres.2006.03.032] [PMID: 16643869]

[97] Choi KT. Botanical characteristics, pharmacological effects and medicinal components of Korean *Panax ginseng* C A Meyer. Acta Pharmacol Sin 2008; 29(9): 1109-18.
[http://dx.doi.org/10.1111/j.1745-7254.2008.00869.x] [PMID: 18718180]

[98] Jiang R, Sun L, Wang Y, *et al.* Chemical composition, and cytotoxic, antioxidant and antibacterial activities of the essential oil from ginseng leaves. Nat Prod Commun 2014; 9(6): 865-8.
[http://dx.doi.org/10.1177/1934578X1400900637] [PMID: 25115102]

[99] Lee KA, Kim WJ, Kim HJ, Kim KT, Paik HD. Antibacterial activity of Ginseng (*Panax ginseng* C. A. Meyer) stems–leaves extract produced by subcritical water extraction. Int J Food Sci 2012; 947-53.
[http://dx.doi.org/10.1111/ijfs.12046]

[100] Zubair M, Rizwan K, Rasool N, Afshan N, Shahid M. Antimicrobial potential of various extract and fractions of leaves of *Solanumnigrum.* Int J Phytomed 2011; 3: 63-7. Corpus ID: 56341364

[101] Parameswari K, Aluru S, Kishori B. *In vitro* antibacterial activity in the extracts of *Solanum nigrum*. Indian Streams Res J 2012; 2(1): 17-31.

[102] Bashir Dar K, Hussain Bhat A, Amin S, *et al.* Evaluation of Antibacterial, Antifungal and Phytochemical Screening of Solanum nigrum. Biochem Anal Biochem 2017; 6(1): 309. [http://dx.doi.org/10.4172/2161-1009.1000309]

[103] Singh A, Mishra A, Chaudhary R, Kumar V. Role of herbal plants in prevention and treatment of parasitic diseases. J Scient Res 2020; 64(1): 50-8. [http://dx.doi.org/10.37398/JSR.2020.640106]

[104] Gupta D, John PP, Pankaj K, Kaushik R, Yadav R. Pharmacological review of Aegle Marmelos Corr. Fruits. IJPSR 2011; 2(8): 2031-6.

[105] Brijesh S, Daswani P, Tetali P, Antia N, Birdi T. Studies on the antidiarrhoeal activity of *Aegle marmelos* unripe fruit: validating its traditional usage. BMC Complement Altern Med 2009; 9(1): 47. [http://dx.doi.org/10.1186/1472-6882-9-47] [PMID: 19930633]

[106] Delgado-Altamirano R, López-Palma RI, Monzote L, *et al.* Chemical Constituents with Leishmanicidal Activity from a Pink-Yellow Cultivar of *Lantana camara* var. *aculeata* (L.) Collected in Central Mexico. Int J Mol Sci 2019; 20(4): 872. [http://dx.doi.org/10.3390/ijms20040872] [PMID: 30781602]

[107] Baba G, Adewumi AAJ, Aina VO. Phytochemical Characterization and *in-vivo* Anti-*Malaria* Activity of *Lantana camara* Leaf Extract. Br J Pharmacol 2011; 2(6): 277-82. Corpus ID: 55140782.

[108] Chekka SV, Mantipelly NK. *Momordica charantia*: A natural medicinal plant. GSC Biological and Pharmaceutical Sciences 2020; 12(2): 129-35. [http://dx.doi.org/10.30574/gscbps.2020.12.2.0251]

[109] Saeed F, Afzaal M, Niaz B, *et al.* Bitter melon (*Momordica charantia*): a natural healthy vegetable. Int J Food Prop 2018; 21(1): 1270-90. [http://dx.doi.org/10.1080/10942912.2018.1446023]

[110] Onyesom I, Onumaechi I, Ehiwario J, Dagana R. Antiplasmodial Activity of *Phyllanthus amarus* Preserves Renal Function in *Plasmodium berghei* Infected Mice. European J Med Plants 2015; 5(1): 109-16. [http://dx.doi.org/10.9734/EJMP/2015/13230]

[111] Onyesom, Onumaechi IF, Ehiwario J, Dagana R. Antiplasmodial Activity of Phyllanthus amarus Preserves Renal Function in Plasmodium berghei Infected Mice. Eur J Med Chem 2015; 5(1): 109-16. [http://dx.doi.org/10.9734/EJMP/2015/13230]

[112] Lee JG, Chae Y, Shin Y, Kim YJ. Chemical composition and antioxidant capacity of black pepper pericarp. Appl Biol Chem 2020; 63(1): 35. [http://dx.doi.org/10.1186/s13765-020-00521-1]

[113] Samuel M, Oliver SV, Coetzee M, Brooke BD. The larvicidal effects of black pepper (Piper nigrum L.) and piperine against insecticide resistant and susceptible strains of Anopheles malaria vector mosquitoes. Parasit Vectors 2016; 9(1): 238. [http://dx.doi.org/10.1186/s13071-016-1521-6] [PMID: 27117913]

[114] Arulmozh S, Mazumder PM, Ashok P, Narayanan LS. Pharmacological activities of Alstonia scholaris linn. (Apocynaceae) - A Review. Pharmacogn Rev 2007; 1(1): 163-70.

[115] Chander V, Aswal JS, Dobhal R, Uniyal DP. A review on Pharmacological potential of Berberine; an active component of Himalayan *Berberis aristata.* J Phytopharmacol 2017; 6(1): 53-65. [http://dx.doi.org/10.31254/phyto.2017.6108]

[116] Chandel S, Bagai U, Semwal RB, Semwal DK. Antiplasmodial activity of aqueous extract of Berberis aristata roots against Plasmodium berghei-infected BALB/c mice. Pharm Biol 2015; 53(12): 1735-40. [PMID: 25858288]

[117] Srinivasan GV, Unnikrishnan KP, Rema Shree AB, Balachandran I. HPLC Estimation of berberine in Tinospora cordifolia and Tinospora sinensis. Indian J Pharm Sci 2008; 70(1): 96-9. [http://dx.doi.org/10.4103/0250-474X.40341] [PMID: 20390090]

[118] Bachani MH. *In vitro* antihelmintic activity of some medicinal plants: a review. IJPSR 2012; 3(9): 3064-75.

[119] Delfin E, Cabardo Jr, Harvie P. Portugaliza. Anthelmintic activity of Moringa oleifera seed aqueous and ethanolic extracts against Haemonchus contortus eggs and third stage larvae. Int J Vet Sci Med 2017; 30-4. [http://dx.doi.org/10.1016/j.ijvsm.2017.02.001]

[120] Kumari S, Kumar P, Khan MA. Sadaf, Husain SA, Singh DK. Anthelminthic/larvicidal activity of some common medicinal plants. Eur J Biol Res 2017; 7(4): 324-36. [http://dx.doi.org/10.5281/zenodo.1036819]

[121] Cala AC, Chagas ACS, Oliveira MCS, *et al. In vitro* anthelmintic effect of *Melia azedarach* L. and *Trichilia claussenii* C. against sheep gastrointestinal nematodes. Exp Parasitol 2012; 130(2): 98-102. [http://dx.doi.org/10.1016/j.exppara.2011.12.011] [PMID: 22209941]

[122] Chattopadhyaya MK, Khare RL. Isolation of anacardic acid from *Semecarpus anacardium* L. and study of its anthelmintic activity. Indian J Pharm 1969; 31: 104-5.

[123] Stepek G, Lowe AE, Buttle DJ, Duce IR, Behnke JM. Anthelmintic action of plant cysteine proteinases against the rodent stomach nematode, *Protospirura muricola*, *in vitro* and *in vivo*. Parasitology 2007; 134(Pt 1): 103-12. [http://dx.doi.org/10.1017/S0031182006001302] [PMID: 17032468]

[124] Thooyavan G, Karthikeyan J. Anthelmintic activity of abutilon indicum leaf extract on sheep tapeworm Moniezia expansa *In vitro*. J Pharmacogn Phytochem 2018; 7(2): 317-21. Corpus ID: 54947647

[125] Binns SE, Hudson J, Merali S, Arnason JT. Antiviral activity of characterized extracts from *echinacea* spp. (Heliantheae: Asteraceae) against *herpes simplex* virus (HSV-I). Planta Med 2002; 68(9): 780-3. [http://dx.doi.org/10.1055/s-2002-34397] [PMID: 12357386]

[126] Erol A, Hamit C, Coşkun H, Turker A, Ozsoy S, Ceylan K. Evaluation of the anthelmintic activity of pumpkin seeds (Cucurbita maxima) in mice naturally infected with Aspiculuris tetraptera. J Pharmacogn Phytother 2015; 7(9): 189-93. [http://dx.doi.org/10.5897/JPP2015.0341]

[127] Md RI, Syeda FTZ, S MIS, *et al.* Evaluation of anthelmintic activity of ethanolic extracts of Carica papaya leaves using Paramphistomum cervi and Haemonchus contortus. Afr J Pharm Pharmacol 2019; 13(12): 146-50. [http://dx.doi.org/10.5897/AJPP2019.5017]

[128] Sahu AK, Panda C, Nayak BS. Determination of phytochemical and anthelmintic activity of rhizome of Zingiber zerumbet. J Pharm Adv Res 2018; 1(9): 399-02.

[129] Choudhary N,Khatik GL, Choudhary SD, Suttee A. *In vitro* anthelmintic activity of Chenopodium album and *in-silico* prediction of mechanistic role on Eisenia foetida. Cell press 2021; 7(1): e05917. [http://dx.doi.org/10.1016/j.heliyon.2021.e05917]

[130] Hudson JB. Applications of the phytomedicine *Echinacea purpurea* (Purple Coneflower) in infectious diseases. J Biomed Biotechnol 2012; 2012769896 [http://dx.doi.org/10.1155/2012/769896] [PMID: 22131823]

[131] Manayi A, Vazirian M, Saeidnia S. *Echinacea purpurea*: Pharmacology, phytochemistry and analysis methods. Pharmacogn Rev 2015; 9(17): 63-72. [http://dx.doi.org/10.4103/0973-7847.156353] [PMID: 26009695]

[132] Pleschka S, Stein M, Schoop R, Hudson JB. Anti-viral properties and mode of action of standardized

Echinacea purpurea extract against highly pathogenic avian influenza virus (H5N1, H7N7) and swine-origin H1N1 (S-OIV). Virol J 2009; 6(1): 197.
[http://dx.doi.org/10.1186/1743-422X-6-197] [PMID: 19912623]

[133] Yang CM, Cheng HY, Lin TC, Chiang LC, Lin CC. Hippomanin A from acetone extract of *Phyllanthus urinaria* inhibited HSV-2 but not HSV-1 infection *in vitro*. Phytother Res 2007; 21(12): 1182-6.
[http://dx.doi.org/10.1002/ptr.2232] [PMID: 17661333]

[134] Du G. Man Xiao, Siman Yu, Mengyi W, Yiqiang X, Shenggang S. *Phyllanthus urinaria*: a potential phytopharmacological source of natural medicine. Int J Clin Exp Med 2018; 11(7): 6509-20. Corpus ID: 84833953

[135] Weber ND, Andersen DO, North JA, Murray BK, Lawson LD, Hughes BG. *In vitro* virucidal effects of *Allium sativum* (garlic) extract and compounds. Planta Med 1992; 58(5): 417-23.
[http://dx.doi.org/10.1055/s-2006-961504] [PMID: 1470664]

[136] Duarte MER, Noseda DG, Noseda MD, Tulio S, Pujol CA, Damonte EB. Inhibitory effect of sulfated galactans from the marine alga *Bostrychia montagnei* on herpes simplex virus replication *in vitro*. Phytomedicine 2001; 8(1): 53-8.
[http://dx.doi.org/10.1078/0944-7113-00007] [PMID: 11292240]

[137] Hayet LE, Gutman L, Aouni M, Maha M. Antiviral activity of *Conyza canadensis* (L.) Cronquist extracts grown in Tunisia. Afr J Biotechnol 2011; 10(45): 9097-100.
[http://dx.doi.org/10.5897/AJB10.2349]

[138] Erdelmeier CA, Cinatl J Jr, Rabenau H, Doerr HW, Biber A, Koch E. Antiviral and antiphlogistic activities of *Hamamelis virginiana* bark. Planta Med 1996; 62(3): 241-5.
[http://dx.doi.org/10.1055/s-2006-957868] [PMID: 8693037]

[139] Cheng HY, Lin TC, Ishimaru K, Yang CM, Wang KC, Lin CC. *In vitro* antiviral activity of prodelphinidin B-2 3,3′-di-O-gallate from *Myrica rubra*. Planta Med 2003; 69(10): 953-6.
[http://dx.doi.org/10.1055/s-2003-45108] [PMID: 14648402]

[140] Kim HK, Lee HK, Shin CG, Huh H. HIV integrase inhibitory activity of Agastache rugosa. Arch Pharm Res 1999; 22(5): 520-3.
[http://dx.doi.org/10.1007/BF02979163] [PMID: 10549582]

[141] César GZJ, Alfonso MGG, Marius MM, *et al.* Inhibition of HIV-1 reverse transcriptase, toxicological and chemical profile of Calophyllum brasiliense extracts from Chiapas, Mexico. Fitoterapia 2011; 82(7): 1027-34.
[http://dx.doi.org/10.1016/j.fitote.2011.06.006] [PMID: 21723379]

[142] Lee-Huang S, Huang PL, Kung HF, *et al.* TAP 29: an anti-human immunodeficiency virus protein from Trichosanthes kirilowii that is nontoxic to intact cells. Proc Natl Acad Sci USA 1991; 88(15): 6570-4.
[http://dx.doi.org/10.1073/pnas.88.15.6570] [PMID: 1713684]

[143] Pu JX, Yang LM, Xiao W-L, *et al.* Compounds from Kadsura heteroclita and related anti-HIV activity. Phytochemistry 2008; 69(5): 1266-72.
[http://dx.doi.org/10.1016/j.phytochem.2007.11.019] [PMID: 18207206]

[144] Wang HX, Ng TB. Examination of lectins, polysaccharopeptide, polysaccharide, alkaloid, coumarin and trypsin inhibitors for inhibitory activity against human immunodeficiency virus reverse transcriptase and glycohydrolases. Planta Med 2001; 67(7): 669-72.
[http://dx.doi.org/10.1055/s-2001-17359] [PMID: 11582548]

[145] Valcheva-Kuzmanova SV, Belcheva A. Current knowledge of Aronia melanocarpa as a medicinal plant. Folia Med (Plovdiv) 2006; 48(2): 11-7.
[PMID: 17408071]

[146] Ooi LSM, Ho WS, Ngai KLK, *et al.* Narcissus tazetta lectin shows strong inhibitory effects against

respiratory syncytial virus, influenza A (H1N1, H3N2, H5N1) and B viruses. J Biosci 2010; 35(1): 95-103.
[http://dx.doi.org/10.1007/s12038-010-0012-8] [PMID: 20413914]

[147] Zhong Y, Zuo C, Li F, *et al.* Chemical constituents of *Phyllanthus urinaria* L. and its antiviral activity against hepatitis B virus. Zhongguo Zhongyao Zazhi 1998; 23(6): 363-364, 384.
[PMID: 11601301]

[148] Hussein EA, Taj-Eldeen AM, Al-Zubairi AS, Elhakimi AS, Al-Dubaie AR. Phytochemical screening, total phenolics and antioxidant and antibacterial activities of callus from *Brassica nigra* L. hypocotyl explants. Int J Pharmacol 2010; 6(4): 464-71.
[http://dx.doi.org/10.3923/ijp.2010.464.471]

[149] Li Y, But PPH, Ooi VEC. Antiviral activity and mode of action of caffeoylquinic acids from Schefflera heptaphylla (L.) Frodin. Antiviral Res 2005; 68(1): 1-9.
[http://dx.doi.org/10.1016/j.antiviral.2005.06.004] [PMID: 16140400]

CHAPTER 5

Exploring the Therapeutic Potential of Medicinal Plants for Rheumatoid Arthritis

Attya Bhatti[1,*], **Ammara Arif**[1] and **Hafiza Ayesha Nawaz**[1]

[1] *Department of Healthcare Biotechnology, Atta-ur-Rahman School of Applied Biosciences, National University of Sciences and Technology, Islamabad, Pakistan*

Abstract: Rheumatoid arthritis is a chronic autoimmune disease that affects the small joints of the feet and hands, causing polyarticular inflammation. Uncontrolled synovial tissue is the most prominent symptom of this disease. If left untreated, it can result in significant impairment, adversely impacting the patient's quality of life and elevating death risk. Genetic, environmental, and epigenetic variables are all important in the etiology of this disease. The risk of developing rheumatoid arthritis is not age-related, people over the age of 40, particularly women, are significantly more likely to get the disease than men. There are a variety of therapies that are provided based on the severity of the ailment. However, all of these therapeutic techniques have negative effects as well as significant prices. More than 80% of the population in the world is now believed to use medicinal plants to maintain their health. Plants are the most abundant source of antimicrobial agents, and extracts of numerous edible plant species, herbs, and spices have long been used to preserve food due to the presence of potentially powerful antibacterial components. Not only minerals and primary metabolites are found in medicinal plants, but also a wide range of possible chemical compounds that aid in the adsorption and neutralization of free radicals. Some of the plants that show antioxidant and anti-inflammatory properties against rheumatoid arthritis are discussed in this chapter.

Keywords: Autoimmune Response, Inflammatory Diseases, Medicinal Plants, Pathophysiology, Rheumatoid Arthritis, Therapeutic Significance.

1. AN INTRODUCTION TO RHEUMATOID ARTHRITIS

Rheumatoid Arthritis (RA) is a disease that is characterized by inflammation of the lining of joints called synovium. It is a symmetrical form of arthritis and may affect multiple joints. Approximately 0.5 to 1% adult population across the globe is affected by it [1]. The disease usually affects the hand and foot joints and takes a chronic manifestation pathway, if not diagnosed and treated early on. The pat-

* **Corresponding author Attya Bhatti:** Department of Healthcare Biotechnology, Atta-ur-Rahman School of Applied Biosciences, National University of Sciences and Technology, Islamabad, Pakistan; E-mail: atbhatti@asab.nust.edu.pk

Atta-ur-Rahman & Ka Bian (Eds.)

ients usually complain of swelling, joint pain, and stiffness. The symptoms overlap with other diseases as well, therefore specific testing and expert clinical consultation is required for accurate diagnosis. The earlier the disease is diagnosed, the better it is to manage. This is because the drugs get a chance to prevent and halt joint damage. If the disease progresses, cartilage loss and bone erosion occur which can be detected radiologically. One of the most important risk factors associated with joint destruction is the presence of autoantibodies [2].

2. CAUSES OF RHEUMATOID ARTHRITIS

Rheumatoid Arthritis is a multifactorial disease, and its onset may be the result of genetic, epigenetic as well as environmental factors. Various whole genome sequencing studies have revealed numerous loci that may increase the risk of RA [3].

2.1. The Interplay of Genes

Multiple genetic loci have been identified in association with the manifestation of this disease. Some of these loci are studied in association with other autoimmune diseases as well. However, inheritance of HLA haplotypes is the most significant genetic predisposition uncovered so far. The HLA-DRB1 alleles code for specific molecules that bear a shared motif of five amino acids. This motif is called the shared epitope (SE). The presence of these alleles causes predisposition to anti-citrullinated protein antibody ACPA-positive RA. Whereas, ACPA-negative version of the disease has been linked to non-SE bearing HLA alleles. One of the examples is HLA-DR3 allele [3].

2.2. Autoimmune Responses Elicited by Posttranslational Modifications of Proteins

When arginine gets post-translationally modified by peptidylarginine deiminase enzymes, citrulline is produced. This process called citrullination is dependent on calcium. Autoantibodies known as anti-citrullinated protein antibodies (ACPAs) are formed against proteins that are citrullinated. These autoantibodies are made by plasma cells in joints that are affected by rheumatoid arthritis. Since, in an inflammatory environment, citrullination of protein takes place, and consequently, ACPAs are generated. An RA synovium may contain various citrullinated proteins. However, the key citrullinated protein found in an RA joint is fibrin [4].

The diagnostic specificity of these autoantibodies is found to be 90 to 95% and they can be identified in 70 to 90% of all patients who are affected with RA [5].

2.3. Involvement of Rheumatoid Factors

Rheumatoid factor (RF) is another major kind of autoantibody that is detected in the serum of patients suffering from RA. It is formed against the Fc part of antibody IgG in humans. It was incorporated in 1987 ACR (American College of Rheumatology) classification criteria for RA. However, ACPA are considered to be comparatively more specific. Several studies have revealed higher disease activity caused as a result of the synergistic effect of RF and ACPA [6].

2.4. Environmental Factors

Tobacco smoke has been associated with increased risk of RA development. Mainly, smoking amplifies the risk of RF or ACPA- positive RA. It causes citrullination of proteins in the lungs. Another interesting observation made by scientists is that tobacco only increases the risk of disease when it is inhaled by the individual. Chewing tobacco does not increase the risk of diseases.

RA development has also been associated with the presence of other inhaled pollutants. These include traffic pollution, nitrogen dioxide (NO_2), silica dust, textile dust and agricultural pesticides.

Another factor constantly associated with the causation of RA is periodontitis. It is a chronic infection of the gums. The risk was almost doubled for incident RA in severe form of this disease that is characterized by the presence of an edentulous state.

Furthermore, a chunk of scientific research has been directed towards finding out the relationship between hormones and RA since RA is known to prevail more in women than in men. In a nutshell, numerous studies conclude that factors that are associated with a decline of estrogen hormone can be termed as risk factors. On the other hand, those that are connected to high exposure to estrogens can be categorized as protective factors [7].

3. PATHOPHYSIOLOGY OF RHEUMATOID ARTHRITIS

The disease onset is due to a combination of genetic and environmental factors. Once initiated, a series of pathological immunological changes snowball into the chronic form of the disease with lethal clinical manifestation.

Endothelial cells play a key part in the inflammatory process initiation [8]. The synovial membrane gets infiltrated by monocytes, T and B cells and neovascularization occurs. Macrophage-like cells and fibroblast-like cells multiply in the synovium. This causes synovial lining to proliferate. As a result, "pannus" is formed. Pannus refers to the expanded synovium. The periarticular bone gets invaded by the expanded synovium at the junction between the bone and the cartilage. As a result of these events, the cartilage starts degrading and the erosion of bone is initiated. Additionally, immune complexes may form that can activate the complement system. All of these processes lead to the stimulation of inflammatory pathways, which are a characteristic feature of RA [9].

4. CURRENT THERAPEUTIC TREATMENTS

The first goal of anti-rheumatic medications is to suppress inflammation and alleviate pain and decrease swellings. Various types of therapeutic drugs are currently being used with different mechanisms of actions. These therapies include NSAIDs, glucocorticoids, DMARDs and biological agents.

4.1. NSAIDs

Nonsteroidal anti-inflammatory drugs are the first choice of drug for RA patients as they act by inhibiting the cyclooxygenase (COX) enzyme which is involved in the regulation of arachidonic acid for the synthesis of proinflammatory prostaglandins. Gastrointestinal anomalies *i.e.*, ulcer, perforation and bleeding and renal complications are the major side-effects of NSAIDs. NSAIDs that act by specifically inhibiting COX-2 are preferred due to lower risk of gastrointestinal abnormalities. Commonly used NASIDs are Valdecoxib, rofecoxib and celecoxib [10].

4.2. Glucocorticoid

Glucocorticoids are a class of corticoids, which act by inhibiting genes causing inflammation in the body. Both genomic and nongenomic mechanisms are responsible for the inhibitory action of glucocorticoids. GCs suppress the differentiation, proliferation, and activation of cells responsible for the synthesis of inflammatory mediators hence, decreasing inflammation. Major side effects of GCs are weight gain, diabetes mellitus, bone-thinning, and suppression of immune system [10].

4.3. DMARDs

Disease modifying anti-rheumatic drugs (DMARDs) are a group of drugs the specifically target molecular pathways responsible for RA pathogenesis. The most commonly used drugs include methotrexate, hydroxychloroquine, sulfasalazine and leflunomide. The potential side effects of DMARDs are oral ulcer, hepatitis, cytopenia, interstitial pneumonitis, cirrhosis, other GI tract complications and hematologic abnormalities [11].

4.4. Biological Agents

Biological agents or biological DMARDs are the latest class of anti-rheumatic treatment that includes biological compounds and immunomodulatory agents. These compounds were introduced after the failure of conventional DMARDs. Biological DMARDs are highly specific than conventional DMARDs and they target specific molecular pathways of RA pathogenesis. This group includes TNF-α inhibitors, IL-1 inhibitors, Anti-β-cell agent, JAK inhibitors and co-stimulation blockers. Several side effects are also reported for biological agents including increased risk of herpes zoster infection, reaction at the site of infusion and production of autoantibodies [10].

All of these medications pose various after-effects and cost issues. These above-mentioned disadvantages related to several anti-rheumatic therapies has caused the shift of drug discovery from conventional molecules to medicinal plants.

5. MEDICINAL PLANTS AND THEIR UNLIMITED POTENTIAL

Human beings have always resorted to nature for fulfilling all their needs. In almost all geographic regions of the world, medicinal plants have been used to cure a plethora of disorders because of their effective therapeutic properties. Scientists have explored the bioactivities of plants and their potential applications for decades.

Plant extracts have been used to derive numerous compounds that have pharmaceutical benefits and play a vital role in treating a variety of ailments. The two biggest benefits of medicinal plants include decreased chances of toxicity and accessibility to the masses.

Different studies have focused on finding a cure for different disorders using medicinal plants. Some of the research conducted, in this regard, emphasizes on cancer, hypertension, heart disease, anxiety, respiratory problems, skin diseases, allergies, infections, diarrhea, stomachache, digestive disorders, migraine, Alzheimer's disease, arthritis *etc.* [12, 13].

6. SIGNIFICANCE OF MEDICINAL PLANTS IN CURING INFLAMMATORY DISEASES

Inflammation is a natural protective response of living organisms to stimuli that might be injurious to them. However, it becomes a cause of concern when the biochemical pathways involved in this process take an uncontrolled trajectory. Hence, the body keeps a strong regulatory check on it. Studies have been carried out to find natural substances that can play an anti-inflammatory role. A number of plants have been identified that exhibit anti-inflammatory and antioxidant activities. Stringent *in vitro* and *in vivo* testing is performed for evaluation of their efficacy.

Sensitive, reliable, and inexpensive bioassays are required for the assessment of anti-inflammatory activity that can detect even minute quantity of a bioactive compound. Once, active compounds are extracted, fractionated, purified from the plant extracts, their chemical structures are studied utilizing various spectroscopic techniques like Mass Spectrometry (MS), MALTI-TOF and Nuclear Magnetic Resonance (NMR), *etc.*

The anti-inflammatory compounds that are identified in plants are chemically categorized into multiple classes. These include terpenes, alkaloids and phenylpropanoids. Phenylpropanoids are further classified into flavonoids, stilbenoids and hydroxycinnamic acids.

Some of the plants with scientifically proven anti-inflammatory activity are mentioned below:

6.1. *Cannabis Sativa*

It contains cannabinoids, flavonoids, and terpenes. Its reported pharmacological activities include anti-inflammatory, antioxidant and antibacterial. Medicinally it is used for reducing chronic pain, nausea, neurological problems, and degenerative disorders.

6.2. *Foeniculum Vulgare*

Its pharmacological activities include antioxidant, anti-inflammatory, and analgesic. The extract of this plant augmented plasma superoxide dismutase and catalase activity.

6.3. *Zingiber Officinale*

Its chemical components include Zingiberene, curcumene, citral and cineol. Pharmacological testing has elucidated its anti-inflammatory activity along with carminative and hypolipidemic properties.

6.4. *Allium Sativum*

The chemical constituents of this plant include ajoene, phytocidin, acrolein, diallyl disulfide and diallyl trisulfide. Pharmacological studies have reported its antioxidant, antimicrobial, digestive and hypotensive properties. *Allium sativum* is also a circulatory stimulant. It is used in the treatment of chest infections, flu, cardiovascular disorders diarrhoea, dysentery, and urinary tract infections.

6.5. *Ammi Majus* Linn.

Chemically, it contains furanocoumarin and bergapten. Its anti-inflammatory activity has been established scientifically. Medicinally, it is used for vitiligo, cancer and AIDs [14].

7. MEDICINAL PLANTS BEING STUDIED FOR THE CURE OF RHEUMATOID ARTHRITIS

Although, a number of synthetic drugs have been recognized to have significant anti-arthritic properties, yet most of these drugs manifest toxic effects. For this reason, scientists have been interested in exploring the herbal medicines for the cure of this disease, since plants are known to be safe when used for therapeutic purposes. Following are a number of plants that have active phytoconstituents and have been evaluated for their antioxidant and anti-inflammatory potential against rheumatoid arthritis.

7.1. *Withania Somnifera*

This plant is a part of the Solanaceae family. It is also called Indian ginseng. It constitutes various bioactive compounds like withaferin A and withanolides. These compounds have exhibited antirheumatic activity in various studies [15].

In one study, conducted on collagen-induced arthritic (CIA) rats, the aqueous extract of this plant showed substantial reduction in inflammation [16].

7.2. *Terminalia Chebula*

It belongs to the family Combrataceae. When phytochemical screening of this plant was conducted, some of the constituents with antirheumatic properties included chebulic acid, sterols, resins and flavonoids [15].

Moreover, hydroalcoholic extract of *Terminalia chebula* exhibited modulatory effect, in the arthritic synovium, on the expression of pro-inflammatory cytokines. Therefore, disease-modifying nature of this plant was established [17].

7.3. *Piper Nigrum*

It is a plant of family Piperaceae and constitutes an active compound called piperine. The anti inflammatory potential of piperine was demonstrated in a study when it caused the inhibition of the expression of MMP13 and IL6. It can either be utilized in a pharmaceutic formulation or as a dietary supplement for the cure of RA [18].

7.4. *Moringa Oleifera*

Moringa oleifera belongs to the Moringaceae family. Its seeds and leaves contain various active constituents such as carotenoids, vitamins, phenolics and flavonoids. These compounds have antioxidant and anti inflammatory attributes. The extract of this plant reduces the severity of arthritis disease. Furthermore, the ethanolic extract of the plant leaves has anti-nociceptive activity. This was shown in a study conducted on Complete Freund's adjuvant (CFA)-induced arthritis rats [19].

7.5. *Curcuma Longa*

The Zingiberaceae family constitutes this plant. Another name for curcumin is turmeric. Turmeric is an Indian spice and an Ayurvedic herb attained from rhizomes of this plant. Some of the names of the active components present in curcumin include cholesterol, campesterol, B sitosterol and stigmasterol. The administration of extract of *Curcuma longa* suppressed the joint and bone degeneration in collagen-induced arthritic rats [20].

7.6. *Coriander Sativum*

It belongs to the Umbelliferae family. Coriander oil has been found to be very beneficial for rheumatism. The antiarthritic activity of hydroalcoholic extract of the seeds of *Coriander sativum* was assessed in adult Wistar rats. Two experimental models were used. These were Complete Freund's adjuvant (CFA) and formaldehyde induced arthritic models. Antiarthritic activity was observed which may be because of the modulation of pro-inflammatory cytokines caused by the extract in the synovium [21].

7.7. *Citrus Limon*

It belongs to the Rutaceae family and is generally known as lemon. The lemon peel extract has multiple bioactive constituents. These include quercetin, pyrogallic acid, eugenol and caffeic acid. Different doses of the lemon peel extract are beneficial for the cure of rheumatoid arthritis. In one of the studies conducted to study its therapeutic properties, it was observed that it caused a reduction in the proliferation of chondrocytes. It also decreased inflammatory cytokines, reactive oxygen species and xanthine oxidase levels [22].

8. FUTURE RESEARCH GOAL

Significant evidence has been gathered regarding the therapeutic properties of medicinal plants, yet very few compounds have been tested and evaluated in clinical trials. It is therefore necessary that advanced studies are conducted to demonstrate the beneficial effects of these plants and their bioactive compounds.

CONCLUSION

There is no doubt in the efficacy of allopathic medicines for the treatment of rheumatoid arthritis. However, to reduce the toxic effects caused by these synthetic drugs, medicinal plants can play a significant role. The bioactive compounds extracted from these plants can be used to make formulations which can be administered as an alternative therapy to decrease the severity of the disease in patients, since numerous plants and their phytoconstituents have exhibited anti-inflammatory and antioxidant properties.

REFERENCES

[1] Firestein GS. Evolving concepts of rheumatoid arthritis. Nature 2003; 423(6937): 356-61. [http://dx.doi.org/10.1038/nature01661] [PMID: 12748655]

[2] van der Woude D, van der Helm-van Mil AHM. Update on the epidemiology, risk factors, and disease outcomes of rheumatoid arthritis. 2018. [http://dx.doi.org/10.1016/j.berh.2018.10.005]

[3] Scherer HU, Häupl T, Burmester GR. The etiology of rheumatoid arthritis. J Autoimmun 2020; 110102400. [http://dx.doi.org/10.1016/j.jaut.2019.102400] [PMID: 31980337]

[4] de Brito Rocha S, Baldo DC, Andrade LEC. Clinical and pathophysiologic relevance of autoantibodies in rheumatoid arthritis. Adv Rheumatol 2019; 59(1): 2. [http://dx.doi.org/10.1186/s42358-018-0042-8] [PMID: 30657101]

[5] Song YW, Kang EH. Autoantibodies in rheumatoid arthritis: rheumatoid factors and anticitrullinated protein antibodies. QJM 2010; 103(3): 139-46. [http://dx.doi.org/10.1093/qjmed/hcp165] [PMID: 19926660]

[6] Derksen VFAM, Huizinga TWJ. Van Der Woude D. The role of autoantibodies in the pathophysiology of rheumatoid arthritis. Semin Immunopathol 2017; 39(4): 437-46. [http://dx.doi.org/10.1007/s00281-017-0627-z]

[7] Alpízar-Rodríguez D, Finckh A. Environmental factors and hormones in the development of rheumatoid arthritis. Semin Immunopathol 2017; 39(4): 461-8. [http://dx.doi.org/10.1007/s00281-017-0624-2] [PMID: 28451785]

[8] Yang XZ, Chang Y, Wei W. Endothelial Dysfunction and Inflammation: Immunity in Rheumatoid Arthritis. Mediators Inflamm. Mediators Inflamm 2016; 2016: 6813016. [http://dx.doi.org/10.1155/2016/6813016]

[9] Hu XX, Wu Y, Zhang J, Wei W. T-cells interact with B cells, dendritic cells, and fibroblast-like synoviocytes as hub-like key cells in rheumatoid arthritis. Int Immunopharmacol 2019; 70: 428-34. [http://dx.doi.org/10.1016/j.intimp.2019.03.008] [PMID: 30856393]

[10] Abbasi M, Mousavi MJ, Jamalzehi S, *et al.* Strategies toward rheumatoid arthritis therapy; the old and the new. J Cell Physiol 2019; 234(7): 10018-31.

[http://dx.doi.org/10.1002/jcp.27860] [PMID: 30536757]

[11] Richez C, Truchetet ME, Kostine M, Schaeverbeke T, Bannwarth B. Efficacy of baricitinib in the treatment of rheumatoid arthritis. Expert Opin Pharmacother 2017; 18(13): 1399-407.https://pubmed.ncbi.nlm.nih.gov/28737053/ [http://dx.doi.org/10.1080/14656566.2017.1359256] [PMID: 28737053]

[12] Dar RA, Shahnawaz M, Qazi PH, Qazi H. General overview of medicinal plants: A review. J Phytopharmacol 2017; 6(6): 349-51. [http://dx.doi.org/10.31254/phyto.2017.6608]

[13] Poddar S, Choudhury S, Chatterjee S, Sarkar T, Ghosh P. Indian traditional medicinal plants: A concise review. Int J Bot Stud 2020; 5(5): 174-90.

[14] Bernstein N, Akram M, Daniyal M, Koltai H, Fridlender M, Gorelick J. Antiinflammatory Potential of Medicinal Plants: A Source for Therapeutic Secondary Metabolites. Advances in Agronomy. Academic Press Inc. 2018; pp. 131-83.

[15] Singh S, Singh TG, Mahajan K, Dhiman S. Medicinal plants used against various inflammatory biomarkers for the management of rheumatoid arthritis. J Pharm Pharmacol 2020; 72(10): 1306-27. [http://dx.doi.org/10.1111/jphp.13326] [PMID: 32812250]

[16] Khan MA, Subramaneyaan M, Arora VK, Banerjee BD, Ahmed RS. Effect of Withania somnifera (Ashwagandha) root extract on amelioration of oxidative stress and autoantibodies production in collagen-induced arthritic rats. J Complement Integr Med 2015; 12(2): 117-25. [http://dx.doi.org/10.1515/jcim-2014-0075] [PMID: 25803089]

[17] Nair V, Singh S, Gupta YK. Anti-arthritic and disease modifying activity of *Terminalia chebula* Retz. in experimental models. J Pharm Pharmacol 2010; 62(12): 1801-6. [http://dx.doi.org/10.1111/j.2042-7158.2010.01193.x] [PMID: 21054408]

[18] Bang JS, Oh DH, Choi HM, *et al.* Anti-inflammatory and antiarthritic effects of piperine in human interleukin 1β-stimulated fibroblast-like synoviocytes and in rat arthritis models. Arthritis Res Ther 2009; 11(2): R49. [http://dx.doi.org/10.1186/ar2662] [PMID: 19327174]

[19] Mahdi HJ, Khan NAK, Asmawi MZ. Bin, Mahmud R, A/L Murugaiyah V. *in vivo* anti-arthritic and anti-nociceptive effects of ethanol extract of Moringa oleifera leaves on complete Freund's adjuvant (CFA)-induced arthritis in rats. Integr Med Res 2018; 7(1): 85-94.https://pubmed.ncbi.nlm.nih.gov/29629295/ [http://dx.doi.org/10.1016/j.imr.2017.11.002] [PMID: 29629295]

[20] Taty Anna K, Elvy Suhana MR, Das S, Faizah O, Hamzaini AH. Anti-inflammatory effect of Curcuma longa (turmeric) on collagen-induced arthritis: an anatomico-radiological study. Clin Ter 2011; 162(3): 201-7. [PMID: 21717043]

[21] Nair V, Singh S, Gupta YK. Evaluation of disease modifying activity of Coriandrum sativum in experimental models. Indian J Med Res 2012; 135(2): 240-5. [PMID: 22446868]

[22] Zou GS, Li SJ, Zheng S, Pan X, Huang Z. Lemon-Peel extract ameliorates rheumatoid arthritis by reducing xanthine oxidase and inflammatory cytokine levels. J Taiwan Inst Chem Eng 2018; 93: 54-62. [http://dx.doi.org/10.1016/j.jtice.2018.07.036]

SUBJECT INDEX

A

B

C

N

O

P

R

S

V

Z

Made in the USA
Las Vegas, NV
12 January 2026

62c10558-46a5-4f3b-8d21-7ab3167f1882R01